GENESIS OF YOGA
Core 26 + Level One

For Fitness, Health and Spiritual Wisdom

Yogananda- Ghosh- Bikram Lineage = Tony Sanchez

1

Tony Sanchez Yoga:
Core 26 + System for Health, Fitness and Spiritual Wisdom.
ISBN: 9798861185462

Photos: Kurt Anderson
Modification photos: Sandra Wong
Text checker: Robert Brain
Graphic designer: Ayelen Di Benedetto

Tony Sanchez Yoga Works
https://tony@tonysanchezyoga.online

CONTENTS

ACKNOWLEDGMENTS

Even though I, never had the pleasure to meet Yogananda personally, his teachings had a great deal to do in shaping my yoga path and for that I am eternally grateful. Through his writings I became aware and a great admirer of his gurus: Swami Sri Yukteswar Giri who he met at the age of 17, Lahiri Mahasaya, Sri Yukteswar's guru and Mahavatar Babaji, Lahiri's guru who introduced him to Kriya Yoga and gave him the mandate to present it to the world. I also felt great gratitude towards Jesus Christ for his teachings, which have revolutionized the world. Yogananda's decision to write his Autobiography and share his knowledge of Yoga, presented itself as a blessing for me, without it I don't think yoga would have crossed my path. I feel this knowledge is indispensable for healing the human spirit, which is an essential part for the recovery of the world as a whole.

I am so thankful for the countless hours Asis (Bikram's older brother) and I spent together talking about yoga and people who have contributed to its development. My special thanks to him for sharing details about Bishnu Ghosh, Bikram's guru and his Hatha Yoga training. And for explaining the difference between Kriya, Hatha, Bhakti, and Jnana, which together formed the eight stages of Raja Yoga and for making me understand their fluid connection.

My admiration and sincere thanks to Bishnu Ghosh for helping modernise old yoga techniques and making important changes in the way Hatha Yoga was been taught and practiced. Bishnu's contribution made it easier for thousands of practitioners around the world to learn, practice and benefit from this great discipline. As a free thinker, Bishnu crossed Yoga techniques with other physical disciplines such as weight lifting and aerobic exercises. His work made him one of the first, if not the first yogi to develop cross training yoga programs and prescriptions based on the students needs to better improve their physical, mental and spiritual health and abilities. Thank you Bishnu Ghosh!!!

And my most heartfelt thanks to Bikram who saw in me the potential to become a committed yogi. And for his trust and time he devoted to my personal training, development and cultivation I will always be grateful. From Bikram I learned Ghosh's Hatha Yoga system and how to combine physical techniques and adopt the exercises to any situation or body type, which is the most effective way to practice this yoga. And I am especially grateful for his strict and demanding training, by enduring it, it made me a stronger, and more flexible, not only physically but mentally as well. Bikram's teachings have reached thousands of students around the world. We owe him our appreciation for making Yoga easier, less mystical and more palatable for the western mindset. By doing so,

Bikram broke a long held barrier and views by Westerners about Yoga, opening the Yoga floodgates and making Yoga all the rage in the Western World.

I am also eternally grateful to Marc Benioff for presenting me with the Zohar "Splendour", The Book of Radiance. This work on Jewish mystical thought known as Kabbalah gave me the greatest understanding on the relationship Yogananda described between Yoga and the world of Jesus Christ.

And my most sincere thanks to Sandy, my wife, for her support, advise and patience. According to her I am not the easiest person to live with, so I thank her for putting up with me all these years. Her work in the field of Yoga, especially Yoga for children, has been most inspiring. And last but not least my gratitude to Steve Delvecchio, Carrie & Shaggy Less Baron, and Amanda Benefiel for reading, and advising me on the content of this manual.

INTRODUCTION

In the Summer of the year 1975, I experienced two major events that changed my life forever: my father's passing (rest in peace) and the lost of my first love "Elisabeth". After those major events my life continued but it was not pretty any more I felt torn inside. At that time I was attending Hollywood High and working at night at a trendy restaurant "The Left Bank" on the Sunset Strip. One day, on my way to work I ran into a friend from school who noticed my sorrow and depression. I mentioned the passing of my father and the end of my relationship with my girlfriend and complained about having problems coping with reality. He looked at me for a moment and took a book out of his back pack, saying that he just finished reading it. Held it in his hands for a short while before handing it over to me, affirming that I should read it. I took the book and glanced at the cover, where a photo of an overweight gentle looking man with long hair and kind eyes was depicted. I read the title out loud, "Autobiography of a Yogi, Paramahansa Yogananda". My friend said he is a yogi from India, I think his message will help you cope better with your situation. I took the book, thanked him, excused myself and on my way, I went.

The following morning after breakfast I started reading Yogananda's biography. I learned about his early life and about his mother's passing which I could relate. His meetings with saints and yogis which he presented as having great abilities and powers, that fascinated me. I could feel and relate to Yogananda's strong, spiritual cravings for "Self Realisation", and the need for a guide which he called a "Guru" to help him navigate through the challenging, spiritual path. What I did not understand was the degree Yogananda was willing to surrender

8

himself to his Guru. Yogananda stated that from the time he found his Guru, he committed his body, mind and soul, giving his Guru complete control over his life. To give oneself to another person, unconditionally the way Yogananda describe his relationship with his guru was foreign to me. For a moment, I thought that maybe if I had given my self to my girlfriend unconditionally, we would still be together. But, no matter, his commitment and devotion toward his spiritual quest were captivating and inspiring.

At the age of 17, Yogananda found his Guru, Swami Sri Yukteswar Giri. An accomplished Kriya yogi and scholar, disciple of Lahiri Mahasaya and Babaji, the so called "Immortal One". Yogananda described his first meeting with Sri Yukteswar, as a divine experience and feeling of profound bliss. At that moment Yogananda said, his pain and spiritual longing disappeared all he felt was a sense of awe and mystery in the presence of the Swami and future Guru. It did not take long before Yogananda and Sri Yukteswar became very close and Yogananda's training on the science of Kriya Yoga began with earnest. Yogananda recalled his lessons been mostly based on ancient Yoga techniques, although they were difficult and challenging, he remembered having done very well to the delight of his Guru. Becoming familiar with Yogananda's Yoga quest, I was beginning to understand the importance of a knowledgeable teacher, guide or Guru, and I wondered if it was possible for me to find a competent "Guru" in Los Angeles, city of Angels.

After months of pain and depression, Yoganada's book gave me a glimpse of hope. I thought, maybe Yoga could help pull me out of the dark mental and emotional place I found myself in. At the same time wondered if I could learn Yoga from a book, if I could not find a knowledgeable teacher or guru, like Yogananda did. As I continued reading, I learned that Yogananda saw the teachings of Jesus Christ and his Yoga philosophy based on the "Bhagavad Gita" as one harmonious basic doctrine. Being Catholic, I had spent my childhood praying with my mom and listening to her stories about Christ, his compassion and kindness. Yogananda's comparison of the Gita to Christ's way was very intriguing for me.

Yogananda described "The path of the yogi" as a moral and ethical path that included compassion and generosity. And from what I understood about Christ, the similarities between his spiritual approach and Yogananda's way were identical. As I read on I learned that Yogananda saw Jesus Christ as one of Babaji's teachers and regular companion creating a strong connection between these two traditions: Christianity in one hand and the Yogic way of the Gita in the other. They both are based on behaviour and purpose meant to heal and elevate humanity to another level of physical, mental and spiritual wellness. At that time, in the 1970s many books were written about Christ but very few books about Yoga were published in America so it was difficult to do an independent comparison. I felt that my best shot to understand the similarities between these two traditions was to emerge in the practice of Yoga, and learn it for myself to be able to make an educated comparison. The challenge was finding a centre were to studied it and practice it.

One day, after school walking down Hollywood Blvd at a distance I saw a group of young people mainly men playing drums, singing and dancing coming towards me. They were singing "Hare Krsna Hare Krsna / Krsna Krsna Hare Hare /Hare Rama Hare Rama / Rama Rama Hare Hare". Their song sounded like a prayer and reminded me of the Christian "chants" sung in monasteries. After the group passed two members lagged behind passing out brochures and other information about Hindu spiritual philosophy. On the front face of the brochure I took was an image of Krishna, above his head the title was written "Krishna Consciousness" and at the bottom of the brochure "The state of awareness in which one acts in complete harmony with the divine or the ultimate reality of Krishna" was written. It was obvious that the Krishna on the brochure I was holding in my hand and the Krishna, Yogananda referred to in his writings were the same deity. I felt a glimpse of hope, I was getting closer to finding out more about this mysterious discipline called "Yoga" and perhaps a place where I could study it.

The next time I saw the Hare Krishna group, I approached a bald young man, dressed in saffron colour garments, smelling like incense. He offered me a translation of the Bhagavad Gita, several brochure and two sticks of incense. I was happy to receive the Gita since I had been looking for a copy for a while but without any success. As I enquired about Yoga classes, he suggested I visited their temple in Venice beach and pointed to the address on one of the brochure. A few moments later, after giving me the information he left in a hurry to catch up with his friends.

The following Saturday, mid-morning I got on the Santa Monica bus and went in search of the Hare Krishna temple. An hour or so later we arrived at the end of the bus's route in Santa Monica beach and the driver pointed me in the directions of Venice beach. I thanked him and got off the bus and started walking. Once I reached the little town I walked all over the place but could not find the temple nor any of the members. I assumed they had already gone to their respective places to sing, dance and preach. After a long while I gave up looking, stopped at a little restaurant close to the beach and had a late lunch before heading back home. A bit disappointed, I have to admit.

Sunday morning I picked up the LA Yellow Pages (phone directory) to look for the nearest Yoga school. This time I was letting my fingers do the walking.

Turning the pages until I found the letter "Y" for Yoga, to my surprise there were only two Yoga listings: Yoga College of India, in Beverly Hills and the Sivananda centre in Marina del Rey. Since I had to work during the week, I made plans to go and check out the Yoga College the following Saturday. I hoped this time would be easier to find the place. That week felt long, I was still emotionally hurting and the days passed painfully slow. I could barely keep my mind on my work. I kept thinking about Yoga and one of Yogananda's quotes "Let my soul smile through my heart, smile through my eyes, that I may scatter rich smiles in sad hearts". Finally, Saturday arrived.

That morning I woke up early, got ready and off I went. I took the bus to Beverly Hills in search of the Yoga College of India. I got off the bus on Beverly Dr, crossed the street and walked down to Wilshire Blvd where the college was located. I did not have to look for it very long, the college was located at the corner of Wilshire and Beverly Dr. I walked through the main entrance of the building and in the far right of the hallway I saw the elevator. I walked over and saw an older man sitting inside it and asked me where I was going. I said, I was looking for the Yoga College of India, "The Yoga College of India is one floor down, hop in and I will take you there," he said. I walked in the elevator, the old man turned a wheel manually to closed the door and pressed the button for the basement. The elevator made several loud noises before it started descending, a few seconds later we arrived at our destination and the elevator stopped. He opened the door, I thanked him and walked out.

I walked into a large reception area, the first thing I noticed were the three large photos hanging on the wall behind a long, tall desk. I was looking at the photo of Yogananda hanging on the right side, when the man behind the desk said "Hello, how may I help you?". I introduced myself and asked for information about the Yoga classes. He gave me his name, "Asis" and handed me a brochure with a photo of a yogi doing a body twisting pose. I turned the brochure over and on the back I saw the schedule of classes listed. The next class is at 10:30 am would you like to join it, Asis asked. I was not prepared to take the class that morning but I could return the following Monday, I responded. I mentioned Yogananda's book and to my surprise his photo is hanging on your wall, I said. Yogananda is Bishnu's older brother and teacher, he said pointing his pen at the photo on the left. Who is the yogi in the middle, I asked. Bikram, my younger brother, the same person on the brochure, he said. My brother was Bishnu's best student and now he is the director and teacher of this college, he said. It was barely past ten when people started arriving for the 10:30 am class. I excused myself and promised Asis I was coming back the following Monday.

I finished reading Yogananda's book that weekend. I was happy that finally I was going to attend a real Yoga class. Monday morning, I got up early and showed up at the college around 8:45 am. I said Hello to Asis, after greeting me he handed me a clipboard with a registration form to fill out. I took it and sat on the long sofa in front of the long desk to filled it out. Once done I stood up, walked over to the desk and returned the clipboard. Asis glanced at the information on the form for a few seconds, then looked at me and said, "If you pay for one class it is 10 Dollars but if you pay for ten classes it will be 70 Dollars, valid for one month".

I only had a 50 Dollar bill and told him I wanted to pay for one class first and decide afterwards if I wanted to continue. "No problem", he said. Took my money and told me he would give me my change after the class. He handed me a towel and showed me where to go. I went into the dressing room, changed my clothes and walked into the exercise room. By that time, the exercise room was almost full of people, mostly women. Some students were standing, others sitting down and a few laying down on their towels, waiting for the class to begin.

A few minutes before 9:00 am Bikram walked in, not very tall in stature but incredibly muscular. His hair was parted on the left side and nicely combed over to the right, leaving his forehead wide open to show his full face. He did not dress anything like Yogananda. His clothes were tight as his chest muscles and biceps were trying to burst out his T Shirt. He was dressed all in white; short sleeve shirt tucked in, polyester pants, big belt buckle and shiny white shoes. In his right hand he was carrying a maroon wallet, it seemed to be full of credit cards and on his left hand his sun glasses and car keys.

Everyone greeted him as he walked in front of the room towards his private dressing area. A few minutes later he came out wearing a tiny black Yoga outfit and stood in front of the class. We all stood up facing him waiting for the class to begin. He spoke for a short while, made some jokes which I did not understand and asked if there were any new students in class. A few people raised their hands, including me. He said not to worry and follow his instructions word for word and that everything was going to be ok. He described the first breathing exercise, then pose after pose for the next hour and a half while we bent, stretched, pushed and twisted our bodies in different forms and ways. The room was hot - about 90 degrees Fahrenheit (32.222 Celsius)- so it did not take very long for most of the students to begin sweating.

At the end of the class, we all laid down on our towels face up in Savasana (Corpse pose). That was the pose I liked the best. I closed my eyes and, then I heard thumping on the wall and suddenly Bikram's voice filled up the room. He sang one of the most beautiful Indian songs. I did not understand a word but the vibrations he created in the room lifted me up and transcended me into another world, something similar to what Yogananda described yogis experience during Samadhi. At the end of the song, we all started to gradually get up and get ready for the day.

I approached Bikram, thanked him for the class and asked about his philosophy on life, he said "Be good to others that others will be good to you". He shook my hand and suggested, I came to class every day for at least two months to get the full benefits of Yoga. He held my hand for a while until I pulled it back and walked away. When I got out into the reception, area and asked Asis for my change he said he did not have it and that I should return the following day with another 20 dollars so I could purchase a card of ten lessons, which I did.

Summer vacation was in full swing and I practiced Yoga every morning and went to work in the afternoons. It took me less than two weeks to do the ten lessons, by then I was feeling so much better that I decided to buy ten more. By the end of the second set of lessons all the morbid feelings I had when I first arrived were gone and I felt great but there was no way I could continue paying for the Yoga classes. So, I told Asis my situation and he said he was going to talk to Bikram about it. The next time I came to class, he said he had spoken to Bikram and they both decided to let me take the classes in exchange for helping them run the desk and do errands when necessary. That was the beginning of a lifelong pursuit and commitment to study, practice, understand and demystify this great discipline called Yoga.

I was very happy to have found the opportunity to learn from a Yoga master so closely related to Yogananda. I started my Yoga practice with earnest and at the same time went back to my father's old Bible to try to understand the oneness Yogananda affirmed between these two great traditions: Christ's Way and Krishna's Yoga. After a short while, it became obvious that the harmonious relationship between Krishna and Christ had to do more with the Jewish Jesus Christ (Yeshua) trained in Kabbalah, the esoteric method and school of thought in Jewish mysticism. And not so much on the Jesus of "The New Testament" based on the four gospels, which were written years after Jesu's death. The New Testament describes Christ's Atonement for the sins of humanity and Crucifixion but nothing about his mystical training.

I read the translation of the Bhagavad Gita I got from the Hare Krishna brother, cover to cover. To my surprise, it was a narrative of a conversation between the Pandava Prince, Arjuna, and his guide and charioteer Lord Krishna right before the Kurukshetra War, also known as the Mahabharata War. A conflict between two groups of cousins, the Kauravas and the Pandavas, for the throne of Hastinapura. The war laid the foundation for the Bhagavad Gita. Arjuna (one of the five Pandava brothers) tells Krishna that he cannot fight his own relatives. In response Krishna explained that it was his duty to fight because of his Dharma or sacred duty which sustains the cosmic order. And as a member of the warrior class he had the obligation and sacred duty of fighting this righteous battle. Arjuna was told to arise with brave heart and push forward to destroy the enemy, and to look at how far he had come rather than how far he had to go. According to Hinduism Dharma is the idea that every person has a purpose (a predestined duty) and is responsible for living out that purpose.

Krishna advised Arjuna that he must follow his own dharma or sacred path to reach fulfilment, implying that it is better to strive on one's own path than to succeed on the path of another. Then Krishna proceeded to presented a set of life lessons about right living outlined on three different Yoga paths: Karma Yoga (path of action), Bhakti Yoga (path of loving devotion) and Jnana Yoga (path of knowledge & self realisation). As I understood, these fundamental Yogas were founded on specific ethical and moral guidelines for "right living" within the philosophy of Raja Yoga. Some of the lessons presented within these Yoga paths included not to be afraid, to concentrate on the work at hand, to do one's very best, and not worry about the results. Also, not to let anger take hold of oneself, to keep control, to have faith and to never run away from personal responsibilities.

Placing the teachings of Krishna side by side with the teachings of Jesus Christ such as "love god, love thy neighbour, forgive others who have wronged you, love thy enemies, ask God for forgiveness, and repentance is essential. I felt that both Krishna as well as Jesus Christ were fighting for the same causes "the soul of humanity" or "right living" but they presented different approaches. I thought that Krishna encourages Arjuna to fight a righteous war as Jesus preached a non-violent approach "Never pay back evil for evil to anyone". I felt a bit bewildered, but I reminded myself of what Yogananda said about Krishna and Jesus Christ, "In the divine plan, Jesus Christ is responsible for the evolution of the West, and Babaji (Krishna), for that of the East". According to Yogananda both Krishna and Jesus Christ are jointly taking care of the spiritual evolution of the world. "In the cosmic plan, the time had come to unite the logical reasoning power of the West with the inner intuitive wisdom of the East".- Yogananda.

In India, Krishna is worshipped as the Supreme God in his own right. He is known as the god of protection, compassion, tenderness and love. And the gospels describe Christ as having two natures: divine and human. In his human nature, Christ experienced all the ordinary limitations and pain humanity suffers with and in his divine nature he is the "Son of God" with many spiritual attributes. Saint Peter, Christ's model disciple and trusted apostle lead the Twelve Apostles in extending the gospels "here and there among them all" (Acts 9:32), including to the non-jewish communities known as "gentiles". Peter was assigned as the rock upon the church of Christ (Catholic Church) was built. In the Gospel of Peter, he addressed the persecution of Christians and strongly encourage his followers to emulate the suffering of Christ. He reminded his followers of Christ's passion, death and resurrection leading to Christ's place at the right side of God. Saint Peter contrasted the divine nature of Christ with the corruption that is in the world and claimed that humanity partakes of Christ's divinity through the promises giving to him and the other apostles by Christ himself. In Peter's agenda were the promises of peace in this world, and eternal life in the world to come by the power of Christ. My feeling is that Saint Peter through the Catholic Church replaced the original teachings of Christ based on the Kabbalah with a more dogmatic philosophical content.

Jesus – Rabbi

While Jesus was never part of the official temple leadership, according to the gospels of Matthew and Mark he was still considered a rabbi because of his ministry. Taking under consideration that between the age of 12 and 30, Jesus life has been unaccounted for, I assumed, he spent that time with the Essenes, a mystic Jewish sect that flourished from the 2nd to the 1st century CE. The Essenes lived in the Qumran plateau located in the Judaea Desert along the Dead Sea. These group of ascetics observed the law of Moses, the sabbath, and ritual purity meticulously. I thought that Perhaps Jesus was educated and ordained as a rabbi during his time with them. Jesus, in speaking to the crowds, proclaimed that he was the giver of the law of Moses and the law was fulfilled in him: "Behold, I say unto you that the law is fulfilled that was given unto Moses". And maybe during the time he spent with the Essenes, Jesus realised he was the "Messiah", the anointed one, saviour and liberator of the world. Another theory about the lost years of Jesus is that he traveled to Egypt and India and came into contact with Buddhism and other Hindu traditions during those years, but there is no historical foundation for this claim.

Learning Jesus's past as a rabbi the Old Testament (Torah) became far more interesting to me. The first book of the Old Testament, the book of Genesis, credited to Moses, is an account of the creation of the world, early history of humanity, and of Israel's ancestors. It states that God made the world and everything in it in six days, and rested on the seventh day. The story goes something like this; "In the beginning (Bereshith) was the Word, and the Word was with God, and the Word was God". - On the first day light was created, "There shall be light, (Genesis 1:3-5) and brought light into existence, before separating light and dark to make day and night". On the second day the sky was created. On the third day dry land, seas, plants and trees were created. On the fourth day the Sun, Moon and stars were created. On the fifth day creatures that live in the sea and creatures that fly were created. On the sixth day animals that live on the land were created and humans were made in the image of God.

On the seventh day God rested, making the seventh day a special holy day.

The first human, Adam was made from "the dust of the ground" and God breathed life into him. Then, Eve was created out of one of Adam's ribs to keep him company and help him and were settled down in a special place created for them called the Garden of Eden. They were made "living souls", denoting living persons. Then God proceeded to bless them, and told them to be fruitful and multiply and gave them dominion over all the other living creatures in the garden. (The biblical view, contrary to contemporary believes of humans having independent souls separated from their bodies, is that humans are living souls). Prior to the first sin, time in the Garden of Eden did not exist, the Living Souls "Eve and Adam" were eternal. They became mortal the moment they disobeyed and ate from the Tree of the Knowledge of Good and Evil. Their action propelled the beginning of time as we know it.

Eating the fruit from the Tree of the Knowledge of Good and Evil caused a rapture between the unchanging, eternal God-the mysterious Ein-Sof (The Infinite One) and the first humans (Adam and Eve). From that moment on they were no longer one with god, they became rivals destined to suffer, struggle and eventually die. Their future generations were condemned to suffer the same fate. As time passed on, the gap between God and the living souls, the first humans got greater, life without the blessings of God became chaotic and challenging. By the time they descended to the earthly, mortal level, Adam and Eve could no longer identify themselves with the divine, their physical bodies and survival demanded most of their attention. On this physical plane, they became part of the finite, material universe God had created and no longer a part of God itself.

Listening to the serpent (Nachash) portrayed in Genesis as a deceptive creature, a trickster, and eating off the Tree of the Knowledge of Good and Evil set off a crucial moment for Adam and Eve. Whether, planned or not, according to the myth, that event was the beginning of the human race, with all its pain, challenges, failures, victories and pleasure. Disobeying God and eating from the tree they were told to stay away from, caused Adam and Eve to begin a physical and psychological downward spiral till they reached the material realm. In this material world, they lost their innocence, learned about sex, had children, multiplied, experienced failure and were fruitful. Once in the material realm, Adam and Eve transmitted to their descendants an imperfect, human nature because of their first sin (sin of disobedience) for that reason all their descendants (humanity) were deprived of the original divinity, justice and wisdom, Adam and Eve knew when they were in the Garden of Eden. Once in the world their physical condition changed, as God had promised they and their children suffered, experienced sickness and eventually death, they became mortal living souls.

Even though the Bible does not use the term Karma, in God's Law of Grace, it presents a similar concept, "You reap what you sow". Contrary to the "Law of Karma", the Catholic Church believes that all can be forgiven by repenting and by the power of God handed down to the disciples of Christ and priest ordained by the church. Wiping out one's sinful behaviour through "confession" we can start with a clean slate as if sins were never committed. In Yogananada's Kriya yoga, we must sow or do good deeds to earn good karma and cancel out bad karma. If you die with surplus bad karma you will have to pay your debt in future lives; there is no mercy in karma, it is pure physics "cause and effect". All in all, in God's Law and in Karma we must be disciplined for our wrongdoings to be mended.

According to Memar Marqa. The teachings of Marqah - De Gruyter, Moses was endowed with an identical glorious body as Adam. "Moses was vested with the form which Adam cast off in the Garden of Eden; and his face shone up to the day of his death."- Memar Marga 5.4. The Adam- Moses connection also looms large in the Rabbinic sources. Even though the gap of time from Adam to Moses has been estimated to be more than 2500 years and from Moses to Jesus Christ around 1500 years, there is a believe that they all met at the Dome of the Rock (Qubbat al-Sakhra), an octagonal structure on an elevated platform in the middle of the Temple Mount in Jerusalem.
This place is revered by most Muslims as the spot from which the Prophet Muhammad ascended to heaven.

The Gospel of Matthew highlights Jesus' importance in Judaism and compares his birth and ministry to Moses' birth and mission: "Jesus is the new Moses who has been appointed by God to free his people from bondage and give the new law".- Matthew 5:17-18. Jesus stated in one of his sermons, "Do not think that I have come to abolish the law or the prophets; I have not come to abolish them but to fulfil them".

The Nestle-Aland Novum Testament Graece, is considered the best authority on Christianity by modern scholars. It declared that there were 76 generations from Adam to Jesus Christ, each averaging around 35 years. From all the passages from the New Testament presented in this text I took the liberty of choosing the ones I considered to be most relevant to Yogananda's teachings: "Anger is a sin if it is without a cause."- Matthew 5:22
"Bless them that course you, do good them that hate you, and pray for them which despitefully use you."- Matthew 5:44
"For thine is the kingdom, and the power, and the glory, for ever, Amen."- Matthew 6:13 "Our Lord Jesus Christ came to call sinners, too repentance."- Matthew 9:13 "For the son of man is come to save that which was lost."- Matthew 18:11 "For many be called, but few chosen."- Matthew 20:22

"Entering into the kingdom of God is hard for them that trust in riches."- Mark 10:24 "We must pray to be ready for Christ's second coming."- Mark 13:33 In the texts the conversation is about "what is good" rather than about Jesus being good and the inference that Jesus must therefore be God."- Matthew 19:16-17 Paramahansa Yogananda (1893-19520) proclaimed that he himself was the "Second Coming of Christ", and was sent by God to the West with the mandate of restoring the teachings of Jesus to their full and original glory. Yogananda left India in 1920 for America, and in the same year gave his first lecture titled "The Science of Religion" at the Congress of Liberal Religions in Boston. During his time in America Yogananda gave over 150 talks and wrote hundreds of articles, many about Jesus Christ's teachings. He run weekly courses, many of which consisted of a half-hour on the teachings of the Bhagavad Gita, and half-hour on the teachings of the Jesus Christ, followed by a discourse demonstrating their fundamental unity. He also published a series of articles based on the teachings of the Bhagavad Gita and another series on the teachings of the Four Gospels in his Self-Realization Magazine.

When Yogananda died, he left a large body of work based on his lectures and seminars along with 30 years of his original writings to be edited. The people he entrusted with this gigantic task compiled and integrated his work into a book titled "The Second Coming of Christ", published in 2004. In the book, Yogananda takes us on a profoundly enriching experience through the Gospels, life, death and resurrection of Christ. He explained a universal path leading to the understanding and realisation of God, never before explained by the different branches of Christianity. He revealed a life-transforming realisation that each of us can experience for ourselves the "Second Coming" by awakening the Divine Consciousness latent within each one of us. He also explained a powerful connection, unifying Kriya Yoga, and the teachings of Jesus Christ. And presented these two disciplines as the foundation to all truthful religions, and I quote "To reveal the harmony and basic oneness of the original Christianity as taught by Jesus Christ and the original Yoga as taught by Babaji (Krishna) and show that these principles of truth are a common scientific foundation of all true religions". - Paramahansa Yogananda

The Ten Sefirot
I studied and practiced Yoga under the tutelage of Bikram and Asis for four years, the last few months of my training I spent at the Ghosh's College of Physical Education in India. And in 1980 I finally got my "Yoga Certificate". During my time at the College, in India, Bishwanath (Bishnu Ghosh's son) was my mentor. After my graduation I returned to the USA, and at the request of Bikram I moved to San Francisco to run the Yoga College of India there. For five years I ran the studio successfully. Around that time Bikram was having financial problems, many times he wouldn't cover my salary which made my

life difficult. Sandy, my girlfriend at that time, started advising me and pointing out all my rights as an employee which did not set well with Bikram. That year on my birthday, Bikram with his accountant drove up to San Francisco and at the end of the day, after the last class ended, I was fired. I was told to get my things and get out. On my way out Bikram approached me and said "no hard feelings, if you ever need anything let me know", and off I went.

I called one of my students, Theo Gund, and told her I was no longer going be teaching at the College of India, and needed help. She said, she was going to ask her husband George, if he could do something about it. A few days later, she contacted me and said that George would help me open my own studio. That took a load off my shoulders, we started looking for a location for the studio, and six months later the San Francisco Yoga Studio came into existence.

During my tenure at the SF Yoga Studio I saw many students in the group classes. I also had a few private students, including Marc Benioff, who was very much into Yoga and Judaism. We had many interesting conversations about the mystical aspects of Yoga in relation to other mystical traditions, especially about Jewish mysticism. One day he presented me with the first three volumes of the Zohar (Book of Radiance) and said that many of the things I had mentioned about Yoga were similar if not the same as the mystical teachings of the Zohar. At the time I had no idea how invaluable these texts were going to be in my spiritual journey.

The Zohar is a foundational work in the literature of Jewish mysticism, known as Kabbalah. It consists on a story about the function of god, the origin and structure of the universe, the creation of souls, redemption, the relationship of the ego to ignorance and finally the connection of the true self in relation to the divinity of God. By comparing the Zohar's narrative to the Yogananda's writings, the Bhagavad Gita and especially to the "Holy Science" written by Yogananda's guru Swami Yukteswar many similarities appeared. In both traditions, the ultimate goal was the understanding of the nature of the universe, manipulation of energy and reunification with the divine. And to reach this level of transcendence and merge with the Godhead the Zohar as well as Yogananda' teachings considered: service, devotion and knowledge essential. In the Gita, Krishna defined these three fundamental human aspects as the three different paths of Yoga: service as Karma Yoga, devotion as Bhakti Yoga and knowledge as Jnana Yoga.

The Zohar tells the departing story of the living souls, and first humans (Adam & Eve) from God and his divine domain (Garden of Eden) to the material world. The story is depicted with ten descending levels, called Sephira (Sephirot Plural), representing the Tree of Life and the Tree of the Knowledge of Good and Evil. The first nine levels form the Tree of Life and the tenth level depicts the Tree of the Knowledge of Good and Evil. These two trees were placed in the middle of the Garden as a symbol of God's life-giving presence, totality of his eternal life and wisdom emanating from himself. After the completion of the Garden, God created Adam and Eve in his own image and set them free to roam among his creation. They were created to "work and serve" in collaboration with God in the ongoing task of upholding and sustaining the order God had established in the cosmos.

The Zohar, in the Sephirotic diagram seem to imply that the essence of Tree of Life and the Tree of the Knowledge of Good and Evil is within Adam and Eve and all their future descendants. This knowledge is considered essential for the salvation of humanity and realisation of God's divine realm. Eating from the Tree of the Knowledge of Good and Evil was the original sin, "sin of disobedience" that led to the fall of the "Living Souls". After they ate the forbidden fruit, God said, "The man has now become like one of us, knowing good and evil. He must not be allowed to reach out hist hand and take also from the Tree of Life and eat, and live fore ever". So God banished him and his companion (Adam and Eve) from the Garden of Eden to work the ground from which he was taken. According to Genesis, this was the beginning of humanity.

The highest level or crown of the Tree of Life is Keter, considered the first and highest Sephira. In this realm, the Living Soul is complete with both positive and negative energies functioning in harmony and endowed with God's absolute light and blessings. As the Living Soul descended, on each lower level it became less divine, denser and more human. By the time it reached the tenth, earthly level the physical body demanded full attention, rapturing the connection to the divine. Once the Living Soul's identification was with the body and no longer with the light of God, out of fear and isolation the "ego" was born, attracting darkness and ignorance. The ego conceptualised the self or I which connected with the external world through perception. It also created a sense of personal identity and feelings of importance which created a bigger separation from the divine experience of unity. In the Sephirotic diagram, the ten descending levels in the Tree of Life are allocated to different parts of the human anatomy with both positive (male) and negative (female) energies.

Sefirot Diagram In Relation To The Human Body
Keter - Crown (brain)
Chokmah - Wisdom (right brain hemisphere, controls the left side of the body)
Binah - Understanding (left brain hemisphere, controls the right side of the body)
Hesed - Kindness and love (right side of the torso, including, arm, hand and fingers)

Gevurah - Strength (left side of the torso, including arm, hand and fingers)

Tiferet - Spirituality, balance, integration, and beauty (spinal column including spinal cord)

Netzah - Perpetuity, victory and endurance (right hip, including leg, foot and toes)

Hod - Majesty, splendour and glory (left hip including leg, foot and toes)

Yesod - Foundation (male reproductive system).

These nine Sephirot constitute the Tree of Life.

Malkuth - Kingdom, this realm is lowest level or emanation on the Sephirotic diagram, associated with the realm of matter, including the earth, and physical world. It is the representation of the material realm, looked upon as being separated and independent from the divine light. This new world is enshroud in darkness and ignorance where the Living Soul is enclosed within the physical body. Originally the only way this physical form (a new living being) could be manifested was through sexual intercourse between male and female (now there is in vitro fertilisation), conception and pregnancy for the "Living Soul" to be born as a living being.

Da'at - Knowledge, this is the place where all the ten Sephirot unite as one, it is known as the "Super Sephira". Da'at represents the "reflection of the inner dimension of the infinity one, Keter", the highest of all the Sephirot. In the Sephirotic configuration Da'at appears along the middle axis, close to the region of the heart, directly beneath Keter. Da'at is associated with the image of God, described as the "One and Only" and it is the location through which the Ein Sof or God prior to any spiritual realm reveals itself. The process through which God, the "Infinity One" reveals itself to create, both the chain-like of spiritual worlds based on the first nine Sephirot, and the physical realm (Malkut) is known as Seder Hishtalshelus. The Tanya an early Hasidic text, states that learning about the Seder Hishtalshelus will bring a person to a "complete opening of the heart".

The divine presence of God in the material world is known as Shekhinah meaning "dwelling" or "settling". This word does not appear in the Bible, it was first used in rabbinic literature. Shekhinah represents the divine feminine attribute of God, associated with the "Holy Spirit", and I quote; "In the imagery of the Kabbalah the Shekhinah is the most overly female Sephira, the last of the ten Sephirot, referred to imaginatively as "the daughter of God". ... The harmonious relationship between the female Shekhinah and the six Sephirot which precede her causes the world itself to be sustained by the flow of divine energy. She is like the moon reflecting the divine light into the world". - Shekhinah is identified with Malkuth, the tenth Sephira representing the material world, she is considered the source of life for humanity on the earthly realm.

Judaism sees Shekhinah as a key, portrayed as a divine winged being dwelling with the people of Israel and sharing in their struggles. It is believe that Moses was the only human considered to have risen beyond Shekhinah into the Sephirotic realm, reaching the level of Tiferet, the sixth Sephira associated with spirituality and balance. Tiferet is known as the bridegroom of the Shekhinah. According to Judaism, God in the form of Shekhinah led the Jews out of Egypt and kept his presence in the Tabernacle as they traveled maintaining a strong connection with them. There is a believe that this connection has continued up to date through worship, primarily worship in the synagogue. There is another theory that the "Tabernacle" symbolises the human being, composed of the body, the soul (mind & emotions), the will and the holy of the holies symbolising the spirit which is always pointed toward and exists exclusively for God.

The Yogic Chakra System
The chakra system is the symbol of the Tree of Life from the yogic perspective. It represents the interconnection of "All Life" creating positive energy and good health when properly balanced. There are seven main Chakras in this representation of the Tree of Life consisting of: Crown (Sahasrara), Third Eye (Ajna), Throat (Vishuddha), Heart (Anahata), Solar Plexus (Manipura), Sacral (Swadhisthana) and Root Chakra (Muladhara) at the base of the spinal column. They hold the body's life energy (prana), but when one or more Chakras are blocked and the energy flow is compromised physical, mental or psychological symptoms such as stress, anxiety, depression, and more can appear. For this Life Energy to remain flowing through them freely, the Chakras must stay open and properly balanced. The fluid flow of this energy will create a harmonious connection between the physical body, soul (mind & emotions), and the spirit.

According to Yogi beliefs, the primary manifestation of Prana (Life Force) is Kundalini-Shakti. I believe that the energy of Kundalini is synonymous with the energy of Shekhinah. From the Yogic perspective Kundalini represents the Cosmic Feminine energy manifesting itself into all forms of matter. And from the Cabalistic perspective, Shekhinah as the daughter of God, and image of the forces of life and mysteries of creation. Yogis believe that, in humans, this Creative Force is found at the base of the spinal column in the "Root Chakra" representing the Earthly Realm in the form of a dormant serpent full of potential energy. In Kabbalah, Shekhinah is affiliated to the tenth Sephira, Malkut associated with the Earthly Realm as well. From Yogic and Cabalistic perspectives, this creative energy or force awaits patiently to be awaken so it can move up through the different energy centres (Chakras - Sephirot) to the Crown Chakra or Keter, the highest realm of the Tree of Life and return to the realm of "Divine Consciousness".

Both, Kundalini-Shakti as Shekhinah are the expression of consciousness and embodiment in the quest for a spiritual connection with the multidimensional cosmos (God). And both seem to follow similar paths which are to ascend from the material realm to the highest expression of the Divine Light. From the Yogic perspective the highest expression of the Divine Light is found in the Crown Chakra in the form of Supreme Consciousness. And from the Kabbalah perspective, it is found in Keter, the highest of all the ten Sephirot found at the top of the Tree of Life. Kudalini-Shakti as well as Shekhinah, they both represent the feminine concept of the expression of God, and they both represent the beginning of the path from the material world to the highest level of Divine Consciousness.

In Yoga, the union of the feminine energy Kundalini with the masculine Divine-Consciousness form one entity, composed of half male and half female known as Ardhanarishvara meaning "The lord whose half is a woman". This entity represents the synthesis of the masculine and feminine energies of the Universe. In Kabbalah, the emanations and characteristics of God are equally masculine (Elohim) and feminine (Shakhinah). Another example of this female-male combination was presented to Moses when God revealed his personal name Yahweh (YHWH) at the burning bush, on the mountain of God, Hored. The name YHWH, consists of a sequence of four consonants: Yod, Heh, Waw, and Heh, known as the tetragrammaton, a combination of both female and male symbols. The first part of God's name "Yah" is feminine and the last part "Weh" is masculine. Another observation, when Yahweh (God) created Adam and Eve, he created them with both male (positive) and female (negative) energies as well, and I quote "So God created man in his own image, in the image of God he created him; male and female created them".

In conclusion, Shekhinah is defined as the "dwelling" or "settling" place of the Divine in the material realm and Kundalini-Shakti is described as the "Serpent Power" residing in the Root Chakra (Earth Chakra) at the base of the human spine. They both are seeing as the "Divine Feminine Energy" and power of creation, and they both are destined to return and reconnect with the highest level of the Divine Light (Supreme Consciousness). In Yoga, this connection takes place in the Crown Chakra (Sahasrara), the highest level of the Chakra's system, located in the head. And in Kabbalah, this connection takes place in Keter (Crown), the highest of the ten Sefirot located at the top of the Tree of Life. In my mind they both represent the same basic spiritual principles. The difference I could perceive is that Kabbalah describes the fall of the "Living Soul" in detail through the ten descending Sephirot or dimensions. But does not give very much information on the ascending process to return to the highest realm. Yoga does not give much information about the fall from the highest realm to the material world, but describes in detail a way back to the "Divine" through the Chakra system in detail. I wondered if the wisdom of the Tree of

Life, Tree of the Knowledge of Good and Evil and the wisdom of the Chakra system originated from the same source of knowledge.

Origins Of A New Philosophy

According to Biblical research, the Book of Genesis suggests that the location of the Garden of Eden was in Southern Mesopotamia, now known as Iraq. During the time of Mesopotamia, around the third millennium BC, trading goods, ideas and philosophical points of view where already taking place between the people of Sumer-Mesopotamia and the people from the Indus Valley.

According to historical records their relationship lasted from 3300 BCE to 1300 BCE. Hinduism started sometime between 2300 BCE and 1500 BCE in the Indus Valley, near modern-day Pakistan. Yoga was incorporated into Hinduism as one of the six major houses of thought in its philosophy.

By the time Abraham, the main character in the Old Testament of the Bible also known as the Torah left Mesopotamia, the communication routes between Sumer and the Indus Valley were well established. According to Biblical records, God (Yahweh) asked Abraham to leave his city Ur Kasdim commonly translated as Ur of the Chaldees, in the early 2nd millennium BC. God promised Abraham land and a long chain of descendants, in exchange for complete devotion and a commitment to the belief in Yahweh as the one and only God. By embracing the "One God belief" Abraham parted ways from the belief in many gods, the way it was traditionally done among all Ancient Civilisations. This new concept (the One God belief) became the foundation for Judaism, Christianity and Islam.

Due to the interconnectivity and exchange of knowledge, and wealth between the Sumerian Civilisation in Mesopotamia and the Indus Valley Civilisation, their philosophical and godly views had many similarities. Unlike the Monotheistic religions that originated from Abraham, Hinduism embraces many gods just like the Sumerians did. Hinduism is considered the world's oldest religion, with roots and customs dating back more than 4,000 years. It is made up of the six orthodox schools that emerged before the start of the Common Era, and some of these schools emerged possibly even before the Buddha. Hinduism has no one founder but is instead a fusion of several beliefs. For many, it's considered a "way of life" or a "family of religions", as opposed to a single, organised religion. For that simple reason, my personal belief is that the beginnings of Hinduism in part were influenced by Sumerians traditions and beliefs. The six orthodox schools based on different world views and teachings emerged in Ancient India way before they were incorporated in Hinduism. These schools or systems (shad-darsana) are as follow: Samkhya, Yoga, Nyaya, Vaisheshika, Mimansa and Vedanta. In Indian tradition, the word used for philosophy is Darshana (viewpoint or perspective), from the Sanskrit root dish (to see, to experience).

1. The Samkhya system, is the oldest of the orthodox philosophical schools. It states that everything, in reality, is derived from "Purusha" meaning the self, soul, or intellect and Prakriti, meaning matter, the creative force and energy.

2. Yoga was incorporated into Hinduism, to help the practitioner on his or her spiritual journey. Yoga represents the loving service to God in the pursuit to Moksha meaning; emancipation, enlightenment, and liberation. Yoga along with Samkhya claim that the only way to reach spiritual freedom (Moksha) is by the separation of the spirit (Purusha) from matter (Prakriti), ignorance and illusion

3. The Nyaya system mixes, both philosophical and religious beliefs. Their aim is to bring an end to human suffering, which originates from ignorance of reality. According to this teachings freedom from suffering can only take place through right knowledge.

4. The Vaisheshika system states that the smallest, indivisible, indestructible part of the world is an atom (anu). It claims that all physical things are a combination of the atoms of earth, water, fire, and air.

5. The Mimansa system is one of the oldest of the six schools in Hiduism. It is based on "reflection" and "critical investigation". This system is fundamental to Vedanta and has profoundly influenced the formulation of Hindu Laws.

6. Vedanta, means the end of the "Vedas". This system reflects ideas that emerged from the study of the "Upanishads", specifically, the study of knowledge and liberation.

Sri Yukteswar, Yogananda's guru, was a renowned scholar, with a profound understanding of the six orthodox schools, the Vedas, Sumerian beliefs, and the Bible. It was Sir Yukteswar the one who encouraged Yogananda to not only learn the yogic philosophy but to study the Bible, and become familiar with Western beliefs. Yogananda had a broad mindset which allowed him to digest his Guru's teachings, and bring clarity and meaning to all the forgotten old traditions his Guru presented to him. Yogananda's uncompromising interpretation of this ancient knowledge was always backed with research, and logical and intelligent wisdom. Deep inside, Yogananda knew his Guru was preparing him to spread the knowledge of Yoga, in combination with the Bible and especially the teachings of Jesus Christ in the West. And to be effective and be able to reach people in the Christian world, he felt he had to be creative and come up with interesting stories to show the similarities of the Bible and Yogic principles for the betterment of the human race.

The following list are some of the most obvious similarities I found between Sumerian Tablets, Genesis, and Hindu Philosophy. They all begin the story of creation, the universe and the human race with the following theories:

1. In the beginning there was chaos.
2. Chaos was transformed to order.
3. God/Gods created all things.
4. Light existed before the creation of the sun and the moon.
5. God/gods were unhappy with humanity and decided to destroy humanity via the flood (Epic of Gilgamesh (Sumerian tablets), Noah (Biblical) and Matsya (Puranas, Hindu).
6. The flood.
7. One man and his family survived the flood.
8. After the flood this man gave thanks to his god.
9. From all of those events; paradise, the concept of eternal life, and enlightenment were developed.

Yogananda's Chakras (7 Energy Centres) & The Tree Of Life (10 Sefirot)
Yogananda depicted the chakra system as seven main focal points related to the five regions of the spine: coccyx, sacrum, lumbar, thoracic and cervical plus the pineal gland (third eye) and the pituitary gland (Crown chakra). Both, the Tree of Life and Tree of the Knowledge of Good and Evil based on the ten Sefirot and the chakra system, based on the seven Chakras are mapped onto the human body. The pathways connecting the Chakras (energy centres), Yogananda called them "nadis". He described them as the playground for the Divine Feminine Energy Kundalini-Shakti found in the Muladhara chakra at the base of the spine in a dormant state. "The awakening and stimulating of this life energy will produce an immense sense of self-awareness and spiritual growth", he said. It is clear that the Kundalini-Shakti and Shekhinah represented the same feminine energy that activates and gives life to the physical body. This Feminine Energy is considered the the Divine Presence of God in the material world.

Yogananda, also referred to the chakras as spinning energy wheels that transmit and receive "Universal life force", through the complex system of channels composed of the network of nadis. He described the Chakras as the seven centres of spiritual power in the human body depicting the precise consciousness level of each individual. According to Yogananda; our personal psychological state as well as our connection to the physical, spiritual and divine worlds depended on the health and purity of these energy centres. He stated, that the first objective in yoga is too detoxify and purify these seven cerebrospinal centres of energy and to open the channels that are spread out throughout the body. He considered this process to be essential to be able to even out and balance the life force within all of us while we are alive, and improve one's health, feel stable, and secure.

Seven Chakras

1. Muladhara - Root (coccyx) Chakra is described as a lotus with four pink or red colour petals, representing the earth and the seat of Kundalini. At this initial level, Kundalini is coiled up with 3 and a half coils in a dormant state. Metaphorically, the first coil wraps around the Supreme Bindu (seed of the universe), the second coil wraps around the Supreme Nada (sound of the universe represented by the syllable "OM"), the third coil wraps around Shakti (life energy) and the half coil connects to the Sakala Shiva (the first of the 7 states of consciousness.) Balancing this chakra creates a solid foundation, allowing the energy of Kundalini to begin the upward flow through the seven chakras to an expanded state of consciousness. When the Root chakra is balanced, the energy of Kundalini produces a sense of stability, confidence, vitality, and strength. The glands associated with this Chakra are the ovaries in women and the testis in men.

2. Svadhisthana - Sacral (sacrum) Chakra, located in the genital region is described as having six vermilion coloured petals, with a white crescent moon depicted in the centre representing the water element. At this level, the energy of Kundalini transforms into a state of fluidity, versatility, and freedom creating a feeling of abundance of creativity and pleasure. This chakra is associated with the the adrenal glands sitting on top of the kidneys.

3. Manipura - Solar plexus (lumbar) Chakra is located between the navel and the breast bone. This Chakra is described as having ten yellow petals, with a triangle inside it, representing the fire element. At this level the energy of Kundalini is transformed into self-esteem and warrior energy, with the power of transformation. It is associated with the gastric gland and it is also responsible for digestion and metabolism.

4. Anahata - Heart & lungs (thoracic) Chakra is described as having twelve smoky coloured petals. Inside this chakra there are two intersecting triangles representing the union of male and female energies. It is associated to the thymus gland and represents the air element. At this level the energy of Kundalini fills the body with love, forgiveness, and compassion, producing a sense of balance, calmness, and serenity. In the Vedic concept this Chakra is associated with the sound of the celestial realm.

5. Vishuddha - Throat (cervical) Chakra is described as having sixteen purple coloured petals. Within this chakra there is a downward pointing triangle

containing a circular white region like the full moon. It is the communication centre of the body and the gateway for the energy of Kundalini to communicate between the lower parts of the body and the head. This Chakra represents space, and is associated with the thyroid and parathyroid glands.

6. Ajna - Third eye (pineal gland) chakra is described as a transparent lotus with two white petals, said to represent the Ida and Pingala channels. This energy centre is a direct link to Brahman, the Universal Consciousness, and is associated with Divine Light. At this level the energy of Kundalini transforms into pure perception, higher realms of consciousness and intuition.

7. Sahasrara - Crown (pituitary gland) Chakra is described as having one thousand petals of different colours. They are arranged in 20 layers, each with approximately 50 petals. At this level the Kundalini (life energy) and Shiva (consciousness) unite, creating a universal flow of energy and spiritual enlightenment.

Yogananda described the chakras as seven occult centres of life and consciousness in the spine and brain, which animate the human physical and astral bodies. He referred to the Chakras as exits or trapdoors through which the soul (Kundalini-Shakti) descended into the body and through which it must reascend through the practice of Yoga and Meditation. According to Yogananda, this is a conscious upward effort by which these seven cerebrospinal centres (Chakras) open and awaken to allow the soul (Kundalini-energy) to freely travel upward to the Crown Chakra at the top of the head. He considered this cerebrospinal pathway to be infinite and the true path by which the soul (represented by the self, mind and emotions) must retrace its course back to God or Divine Consciousness.

When Yogananda arrived in the West, he introduced his brand of Yoga as Kriya Yoga. In the Bhagavad Gita this Yoga is featured as Karma Yoga or Yoga of service. Yogananda presented it as the first step of the Royal Path to help cleanse and purify the Chakras (energy centres) and connecting Nadis (energy channels) in the body to improve the overall circulation of energy. The two fundamental parts of Kriya Yoga are based on a system of observances and ethical rules for Right Living: the Yamas and Niyamas. They are the first two branches of Patanjali's Ashtanga Yoga (Eight limb Yoga), also known as Raja (Royal) Yoga. The Yamas are five observances: nonviolence, truthfulness, not stealing, moderation of the senses, and non-greed. And the Niyamas are five ethical rules: purity, contentment, self-discipline, self-study, and surrendering to God. Yogananda combined the Yamas, Niyamas and the Ten Commandments creating a system for right living that was easy for Westerners to accept. The Ten Commandments also known as the Law of Moses, Jesus Christ proclaimed to be the giver and representative of this law. By embracing and making the

Ten Commandments part of Kriya Yoga, Yogananda was able to find great acceptance in the Christian World.

By incorporating the Ten Commandments into the fold of Kriya Yoga, Yogananda open the doors for many Christians in the West to dabble in the mysterious philosophy of the yogis. The Ten Commandments, the Yamas and the Niyamas, were present by Yogananda as essential for the ascension of the soul to the highest realm of Divine Consciousness represented by the Crown Chakra in the Yoga tradition and Keter, the highest Sephira at the top of the Tree of Life in the Kabbalah tradition.

Ten Commandments:
1. You shall have no other gods before me
2. You shall not make idols
3. You shall not take the name of the Lord your God in vain
4. Remember the Sabbath day, to keep it holy
5. Honour your father and your mother
6. You shall not murder
7. You shall not commit adultery
8. You shall not steal
9. You shall not bear false witness against your neighbour
10. You shall not covet

Yamas:
11. Ahimsa - non-violence
12. Satya - truthfulness
13. Asteya - non-stealing
14. Brahmacharia - moderation
15. Aparigraga - non-hoarding

Niyamas:
1. Saucha - purity
2. Santosha - contentment
3. Tapas - austerities
4. Svadhyaya - self study
5. Ishvara - surrender to the higher source

Raja (Royal) Yoga / Tree of Yoga
The meaning of Yoga in Sanskrit is "Yoking" or "Union". Yoga is the second of the six schools "Darshan" in the Hindu Philosophy. This Darshan (school) is based on the "The Yoga-Sutras of Patanjali", which were very much influenced by the philosophy of Samkhya, the first of the six schools of Hindu Philosophy. It is speculated that the Sutras were arranged between the 2nd Century BC

and the 5th Century AD. This arrangement consisted of four different texts: "Psychic Power", "Practice Yoga", "Samadhi" (a state of intense concentration leading to divine consciousness), and "Kaivalya" (Detachment of the spirit from matter). These ancient texts, together feature 195 aphorisms (Sutras). The Sutras presented Yoga as a practical approach for physical purification and mental health, complemented by the more intellectual Samkhya content consisting on the dualistic view of matter (prakriti) and the eternal spirit (Purusha).

These two systems: Yoga and Samkhya advocated that the attainment of spiritual freedom (moksha) could only happen when the spirit (purusha) is disengaged from the bondage of matter (prakriti), ignorance and illusion. Their combine view of the downward evolution from the Divine to the Material Realm is the same as the view of the downward spiral presented by the Tree of Life and the Tree of the Knowledge of Good and Evil in the Sephirot system from Kabbalah. The mission presented by Yoga, Samkhya, the Chakra system and Kabbalah is to purify the Self, and reverse the downward cycle of the human condition. The four systems follow a similar process intended to lead the Self back to its original state of purity to be able to reenter the Divine Realm. It is essential to learned how to control and suppress the toxic and negative activities of the mind to be able to succeeded in ending attachment to material objects and be able to enter Samadhi, a state of deep concentration that results in a blissful elated union with the ultimate reality.

The eight stages or limbs of Raja Yoga, described by Patanjali in his Sutras, present different facets of how to embody mental, physical and spiritual unity. The first two stages are ethical preparations: Yama (restraint), which denotes abstinence from injury, falsehood, stealing, lust, and avarice; and Niyama (discipline), which denotes purification of the body and mind, contentment, austerity, study, and devotion to God. The next two stages or limbs: Asana (seat) and Pranayama (breath control) are for physical and mental preparation. Asana (Yoga postures) help condition the body, making it supple, flexible and healthy. And Pranayama (breath control), based on a series of breathing exercises is intended to stabilise the rhythm of the breath in order to develop respiratory and mental relaxation. The fifth stage is Pratyahara (withdrawal of the senses). This technique is based on managing the senses by concentrating them inwardly, in order to control the mind.

Whereas the first five stages or limbs are external practices, the remaining three are purely mental or internal techniques. The sixth stage or limb is Dharana (fixed attention) is the active focusing and concentration on one point without wavering. The seventh stage or limb is Dhyana (concentrated meditation) is the uninterrupted contemplation of the object of meditation, beyond any memory of ego. The final stage or limb is Samadhi (total self-collectedness) is a precondition of attaining freedom from samsara, or the cycle of rebirth. In this stage the meditator perceives or experiences the object of his meditation and himself as one.

These eight Yoga stages act as guidelines on how to live a meaningful and purposeful life. When divided, they form the four Classical Paths of Yoga: Karma also known as Kriya Yoga, Hatha Yoga, Bhakti Yoga, and Jnana Yoga, together they form Raja Yoga (The Royal Path). Their unified objective is to train the practitioner to self observe and become aware of his or her nature to cultivate discernment, awareness, self-regulation and higher, divine consciousness. These four paths: Karma, Hatha, Bhakti and Jnana presented as Raja Yoga (Royal Yoga) form the second Darshan (School) in Hindu philosophy. They all originated from the same source and resting place, and are the representation of the four branches of the Yoga Tree.

1. Karma Yoga (Yoga of service) is based on first two Yoga Limbs: Yama (restraint) and Niyama (discipline). Yogananda presented this Yoga to the Western world as Kriya Yoga.

2. Hatha Yoga (Yoga for health) is based on the third and fourth Yoga Limbs: Asana (Yoga postures) and Pranayama (breath control). The original asanas were sedentary positions for controlling the breath and for meditation. Around the 10th century AD, Matsyendranah (creator of Hatha Yoga) expanded these sitting positions and breathing techniques into more active and therapeutic poses and breathing exercises. From this time on the health of the body became an important prerequisite in Yoga for spiritual development. Later on, many other exercises from gymnastics, dance and martial arts were incorporated into the Hatha Yoga fold. Bishnu Ghosh, Yogananda's younger brother, expanded on the Hatha Yoga Pradipika knowledge to developed his own unique brand of Hatha Yoga.

3. Bhakti Yoga (Yoga of devotion) is based on the fifth and sixth Yoga Limbs: Pratyahara (withdrawal of the senses) and Dharana (concentration). This Yoga is a spiritual path focused on loving devotion towards God and towards the development of one's personal divinity. Most organised religions have adopted this approach.

4. Jnana Yoga (Yoga of knowledge) is based on the seventh and eighth Yoga Limbs: Dhyana (meditation) and Samadhi (absorption). This yoga is one of the classical paths in Hinduism, which emphasises the "Path of knowledge", also known as the "Path of Self-realisation"

These four styles of yoga can be practice individually or as one progressive path. Each one deals with specific aspects of the human being (body-mind-emotions system), for example: Karma Yoga deals with the active aspect of the mind and it is considered the great purifier. Hatha Yoga deals with physical and mental health as preparation for the more advanced aspects of Yoga. Bhakti Yoga deals with the emotional aspect and it is based on loving recollection of God and the self. Most religions adopted this spiritual path because is considered the most natural. And Jnana Yoga deals with the intellectual aspect of the human being. Jnana's fundamental goal is to liberate the mind from the illusionary world of Maya (negative self-limiting thoughts and perceptions) and to unite the inner-Self (Atman) with the Oneness of all life, the Brahman.

The Materialisation Of The Soul

For a better understanding of the nature of the humans soul, we must first go back to when our first ancestors appeared. According to the latest anthropological studies, this phenomenon took place between six and seven million years ago, probably our oldest relatives were ape like creatures in Africa. The six plus million years we (humans) have been on Earth have allowed us to evolve, build tools, create civilisations, adapt to our environment, organise religions and become the humans we are today. In the course of human evolution, the practice of living in a group with mutual understanding and dependency became very useful and a practical life style, and from small isolated groups, larger communities formed. After that came societies, which in time became civilisations and through it all we created rituals honouring and commemorating the dead. Therefore the idea of a human soul and the afterlife was conceptualised within a dimensional universe.

OLDEST CIVILISATION

The oldest known Civilisation as far as we know was "Sumer" in Mesopotamia. It was the first Civilisation to identified the human soul as a transient entity that moves to the underworld after the body dies. Research and studies on this ancient Civilisation has shown that they defined the underworld as the cosmic opposite of the heavens and life on earth. The origin of this Civilisation dates back so far that there is no evidence of any other civilised society before them. The pinnacle of their power was from about 3500 BCE - 500 BCE in the current location of Iraq, Syria and Turkey.

The Bible, capitalised on the knowledge of the Sumerians, refined it and was presented by Abrahamcas as the New World Order, ordained by God. Abraham was a native of Ur, the ancient city in Mesopotamia. The story goes more or less as it follows: "One day God (Yahweh) called on Abraham and promised to make him the father of great nations, to guide him and protect him in exchange for his loyalty." Apparently, this was the break away from the old Sumerian beliefs based on the worship of many gods and the beginning of a new concept, consolidating all worship to one God (Yahweh). By the end of the Babylonian Captivity (6th century BCE), the very existence of other Gods was denied, and Yahweh was proclaimed as the creator of the cosmos, the one true universal God, omnipotent, omnipresent with the power to intervene in the world of humans.

Abraham was 100 years old when his wife Sara gave birth to his second son Isaac. Though he was Abraham's second child it was Sarah's only child and inheritor of his father's blessings. Isaac founded Israel and became an important figure in Christianity as well. Apparently, the genealogy of Jesus is traced back to Isaac. Abraham's first son Ishmael was born to Sarah's Egyptian handmaiden Hagar. In Islam, Ishmael is regarded as a prophet and ancestor to Muhammad.

Abraham became the father, patriarch of the three major monotheistic religions: Judaism, Christianity and Islam. The three religions embraced the belief that every human being has an individual "soul" that needs redemption contrary to the Bible's description. The Bible calls the soul "Nephesh" meaning "Living Soul" in Hebrew, and makes reference to a living, breathing conscious body, rather than an immortal soul. This living, breathing body-soul (human being) is endowed with two fundamental elements: the contemplative and the active. I believe these two fundamental elements are parts of the parasympathetic (contemplative-mental) and the sympathetic (active- physical) nervous systems.

The parasympathetic system consists on the cranial nerves and is considered the contemplative part of the Human being. This system controls the senses and the intellect and is considered the higher part of the Human-Being. And the sympathetic nervous system based on the spinal nerves is responsible for controlling all physical functions and body movements. This system allow us to descend and actively participate in the for ever changing material world. This physical participation (actions-karma/ energy manipulation) within the world helps craft our individual personalities which are considered the lower part of the Living-Being. The material, external world and the internal spiritual realm are two dimensions of the Human Being and should work together for better physical and spiritual development.

Society, family responsibilities and personal needs and wants demand activity and toil in the material world which makes us denser, more rigid and stressed. On the other hand, inner spiritual practices such as prayer, meditation and Yoga help raise the vibrations of the Living Being (Living- Soul) and evolve into higher and higher frequencies of being. In my view, these frequencies depend on the health and condition of the parasympathetic and sympathetic nervous systems. When properly nurture and trained, these two systems will help us break the bounds limiting or preventing us from living within infinity.

SECOND OLDEST CIVILISATION

The second oldest civilisation recorded is the civilisation of the Indus Valley in the Northwestern regions of South Asia, lasting from 3300 BCE to 1300 BCE. Indus-Mesopotamia relations are estimated to have taken place from the 3rd millennium BCE to 1900 BCE when the Indus Valley Civilisation ended. The war leading to their destruction is told in the Rig Veda, the earliest of the four Vedas and one of the most important texts in Hinduism. This collection of hymns (the Vedas) in praise of the Gods, (not a monotheistic concept) were written by the Rishis also known as the Siddhars a group of holy men in the late Harappa period. These scriptures are guidelines for daily living as well as religious rituals, family and society norms. Another major epic written around the same period of time was the Mahabharata.

The most famous part of the Mahabharata is the Bhagavad Gita (written some time between 400 BCE and 200 CE) which gives an account of the Kurukshetra war. The Gita is based on the conversation between Krishna and Arjuna on the battle field while Arjuna waited for fighting to begin. There is a hypothesis that Lord Krishna lived 2000 years before the Indus Valley Civilisation existed. This is according to discoveries made by archeologists at the submerged city of Dwarka off the coast of the Western state of Gujarat in India. Therefore Arjuna's conversation with Krishna took place in a vision described in chapter 11 of the Bhagavad Gita.

Arjuna said:

My Lord! Your words concerning the Supreme Secret of the Self, given for my blessings, have dispelled the illusion which surround me.

Oh Lord! Whose eyes are like the lotus petal! You have described in detail the origin and the dissolution of being, and Your own Eternal Majesty.

I believe all as You have declared it. I long now to have a vision of Your Divine Form, O you Most High!

If You think that it can remade possible for me to see it, show Me, O Lord of Lords! Your own Eternal Self.

Lord Krishna replied:

Behold, O Arjuna! My celestial forms, by hundreds and thousands, various in kind, in colour, and in shape.

Behold the powers of nature: fire, earth, wind, and sky; the sun, the heavens, the moon, the stars; all the forces of vitality and healing; and the moving winds. See the myriad wonders revealed to none but you.

Here, in Me living as one, O Arjuna! Behold the whole universe, movable and immovable, and anything else that you would see.

Yet since with mortal eyes you cannot see me, lo! I give you Divine Sight. See now the glory of my Sovereignty.

Having thus spoken, Lord Krishna, the Almighty Prince of wisdom, showed to Arjuna his Supreme Form.

During this conversation, Krishna points out that all wars first exist in the mind. And thus winning in the mind is the first step to winning on the battlefield and in real life. Krishna, also revealed the secret knowledge of three fundamental yogic paths:

According to the narrative, Arjuna saw Krishna as a Supreme Being, the source of awe and wonder with the splendour of a thousand suns. In his vision, Arjuna received the knowledge of the Bhagavad Gita "Song of God" and was advised about the fighting that was about to take place. Lord Krishna invoked the concept of dharma (sacred duty), a cosmic law underlying right behaviour and social order sustaining the cosmos as the reason for this battle. According to the caste system, dharma differs based on the class and caste into which a person is born. As a member of the warrior class Arjuna had the primary sacred duty of fighting this righteous battle.

According to the narrative, Arjuna stood behind Krishna inside the spoked wheel Chariot, pulled by five horses. The Chariot was a gift of Agni, the fire God to Arjuna. This Chariot could be controlled and dominate all directions in any terrane including in the three worlds: heaven, earth and the netherworld. The Chariot was named "Nandi Ghosh" and the Chariot's flag was called "Kapi Dhvaja", which had the figure of Hanuman (the monkey God) depicted on it. Metaphorically, the Chariot represents the human body and the horses the five senses: smell, taste, sight, hearing and touch. The chariot's reins, which the charioteer (Krishna) used to drive the Chariot, symbolises the human mind. The Charioteer or driver represents human intelligence and the passenger (Arjuna) symbolises the human spirit or soul.

INDUS VALLEY CIVILISATION AND THE SIDDHARS

The first group of adepts, followers of Shiva in the Indus Valley were known as the Siddhars also known as Rishis or Yogis. They considered Lord Shiva to be the first Yogi and the first God which communicated to them sacred sounds and texts after intense meditation. This knowledge was originally transmitted orally, in the form of the Four Vedas (2nd millennium BCE.) The Siddhars also created a system of medicine based on a combination of ancient medicinal practices, sitting positions, breathing exercises, meditation, spiritual rituals, alchemy and mysticism. Some of these disciplines eventually became the roots of Yoga. The Siddhars were considered masters of the "ashta-siddhis", eight supernatural, psychic and magical powers:

> Anima - the ability to perceive the microscopic world.
> Mahima - the ability to see the structures of the galaxies.
> Garima - the power to become infinitely heavy at will.
> Laghima - the power to become weightless, lighter than air.
> Prapti - the power to instantaneously travel or be anywhere at will.
> Prakamya - the power to assume any shape or form at will.
> Isitva - the power to become very small.
> Vasita - the power to control the material world including Maya, also known as human illusion.

In the Eight Limbs of Yoga Patanjali, one of the original Siddhars points out to dharana, dhyana and samadhi are the principle techniques to gain full control of the eight (siddhis) powers.

THE DOWNWARD SPIRAL OF THE SOUL

The book of Genesis is the first book of the Torah and of the Christian Old Testament. It depicts the account of the creation of the cosmos and the early history of humanity accredited to the Biblical God Yahweh (YHWH). The same god to whom Jesus prayed. The name YHWH, consisting of the sequence of letters: Yod, Heh, Waw and Heh, is known as the tetragrammaton. It is the occult key that unlocks the meaning behind astrology, Bible and Kabbalah mysteries. This include elements incorporated within the conception and understanding of the Tree of Life and Tree of the Good and Evil (ten Sefirot), the divine essence of God, the ten commandments, and the feminine element of the Godhead.

In the beginning (Beresheet) - "God created the heavens and the earth, and the earth was without form, and void; and darkness was upon the face of the deep. And the Spirit of God moved upon the face of the waters". God (Yahweh), completed creation with all its wonders in six days and on the seventh day, he rested and blessed the day as the holy "Sabbath." "By the word of God the heavens were made, their starry host by the breath of his mouth" (Psalm 33:6)

Day One
On the first day God said, "Let there be light; and there was light" Genesis 1:3. God began the process of creation by extending himself as the Adam Kadmon within the void (space) manifested for creation to take place. On the first day, God separated the light from the dark creating day and night. Adam Kadmon also called Elyon, or Adam lla'ah, is the first of the Four Worlds that came into

being after the contraction of God's infinite light.

Day Two
On the second day, God created the firmament. "Let there be an expanse in the midst of the waters (void-space), and let it separate the waters that where under the expanse from the waters above the expanse. And it was so. And God called the expanse Heaven. And there was evening and there was morning, the second day (Genesis 1:6-8). On the second day the firmament separated the earth from the heavens.

Day Three
On the third day, God separated the land from the waters and created vegetation. These acts were created for the continuance of life. The waters gathered together, God called them Seas; and within each form of vegetation he put seeds, each according to its kind."

Day Four
On the fourth day, God created the sun, moon, and stars after he created light. "Let there be lights in the expanse of the heavens to separate day from night. And let them be for signs and for seasons, and for days and years, and let them be lights in the expanse of the heavens to give light upon earth." "And it was so, And God made the two great lights - the greater light to rule the day and the lesser light to rule the night - and the stars. And God set them in the expanse of the heavens to give light on the earth, to rule over day and over night, and to separate the light from the darkness". (Genesis 1:14-18).

Day Five
On the fifth day, God created more life. "Let the waters swarm with swarms of living creatures, and let birds fly above the earth across the expanse of the heavens." "After creating all the living creatures in the seas and every winged bird on the face of the earth God blessed them; Be fruitful and multiply and fill the waters in the seas, and let birds multiply on the earth" (Genesis 1:20-22).

Day Six
On the sixth day, "God created other animals including, every creature that creeps on the ground". Then God said, "Let us make man in our image, after our likeness. And let them have dominion over the fish of the sea and over the birds of the heavens and over the livestock and over all the earth and over every creeping thing that creeps on the earth" (Genesis 1:26).

By creating man (Adam & Eve) on his own image, God placed humanity only second to him. They were blessed and given the following decree; "Be fruitful and multiply and fill the earth and subdue it, and have dominion over the fish of the sea and over the birds of the heavens and over every living thing that moves on the earth." And God said, "Behold, I have given you every plant yielding seed that is on the face of all the earth, and every tree with seed in its fruit. You shall have them for food." (Genesis 1:28-9).

Day Seven

On the seventh day, God decreed the entirety of his creation as "Very Good" and rested, not because he was tired but because he wanted to set aside that time for a relationship with his creation. God blessed and sanctified the seventh day as a mark and a sign of his sovereignty as Creator of the heavens and the earth.

Yahweh (YHWH) made man (Adam) of the dust off the ground and breathed into his nostrils the breath of life; and Adam became a "Living Soul". The breath of life placed in the lifeless body of man in Kabbalah is known as the primordial spirit named Adam Kadmon. The primordial spirit originated from the first spiritual world that came into being after God contracted his infinite light. By contracting his infinite light (Ohr Ein Sof) and placing it in the body of man, God didn't only give him life but gave him mind and the power to think. Adam was endowed with a big, complexed brain big enough for his mind to grow, evolved and develop conceptual knowledge.

The primordial spirit (Adam Kadmon) breathed into the lifeless body of Adam, gave him life and animated him before the mind, intellect and senses came to be. Once man had a body, mind and divine life, God was satisfied and let him be. Man (Adam) had the whole Garden of Eden for himself, but was lonely. One day, after seeing Adam all alone, wondering in the garden, God felt a bit sorry for him. And to take care of this issue, one night while Adam slept God made a woman (Eve) from one of his ribs. God wanted the couple to live as a husband and wife in the Garden of Eden among all the other creatures God had already created. The Garden of Eden was there for them to enjoy, guard and named everything in it. They were also told they could eat from all the fruit trees except from the Tree of Knowledge of Good and Evil and the Tree of Life both located in the centre of the garden.

They were happy, everything was just perfect, until one morning as the woman (Eve) walked near the Tree of the Knowledge of Good and Evil a speaking serpent addressed her and suggested she eat the fruit from the forbidden tree. In response the woman said; "We may eat off the fruit of the trees in the garden; but God said, "you shall not eat off the fruit of the trees that are in the middle of the garden, nor shall you touch them, or you shall die". Genesis 3:2-3.

The serpent replied that she would not surely die (Genesis 3:) but if she ate the fruit of the tree, the serpent said, "then your eyes shall be opened, and ye shall

be as gods, knowing good and evil." "Eve, ate the fruit and brought some to Adam and he also ate." Their divinity and innocence at that moment died and the mixture of good and evil became part of their daily lives. Creation took a different route from the originally plan God had envisioned or did it? That is the question most scholars wrestle with. After eating off the Tree of the Good and Evil "Their eyes were opened and they knew they were naked and sewed fig leaves together, and made themselves aprons." Later that afternoon, "They heard the voice of the LORD God walking in the garden in the cool of the day; and Adam, his wife and the snake hid themselves from the presence of the LORD God amongst the trees of the garden." And LORD God said "Behold, the man is become as one of us, to know Good and evil: and now, lest he put forth his hand, and take also of the tree of life, and eat, and live for ever." 3:23: When Adam and Eve finally came out of their hiding place, looking frighten and guilty, God looked at them and demanded an explanation. It is a popular believe that their disobedience caused God's anger which created ripples and disorder in creation. And humanity inherited sin and guilt not because Eve and Adam eat the apple but because they disobeyed God. My feeling is that, after braking their promise God wanted them to own up, admit their disobedience and take responsibility. Which of course they did not, instead they blame each other. They were the first humans after all.
Covering up the sin became worse than the sin itself.

Adam blamed Eve and Eve blamed the Serpent, and in his disappointment, God with a thunderous voice declared to Adam; "Because you listened to your wife and ate from the tree about which I commanded you, "You must not eat of it", by the sweat of your face you shall eat bread, till you return to the ground, for out of it you were taken; for you are dust and to dust you shall return." I think the curse Adam received is a metaphor for the difficulties of agriculture, the hard work of planting, harvesting and working the land, the beginning of the Agricultural Age. The second curse was to Eve; she would endure pain and suffering in bearing children. And thirdly God said to the serpent; "Because you have done this. "cursed are you above all livestock and all wild animals! You will crawl on your belly and you will eat dust all the days of your life".

God spelled them from the garden and to ensure that they did not return and eat from the Tree of Life and live for ever, God placed two cherubim at the east end of the Garden to guard and protect the path to the tree. Outside the garden, Adam and Eve were no longer divine nor protected from the Law of Cause and Effect (Law of Karma). As humans, probably without realising it, Adam and Eve set of a number of consequences in the process of creation that eventually became the 12 laws of Karma:

> The Great Law or the Law of Cause and Effect. This is a universal law, it specifies that every single action in the universe produces a

reaction meaning "every action has an equal and opposite reaction". Even human though creates movement and a reaction no matter how minute it is.

The Law of Creation; this law states that the force of the creation energies and activation is inherent in all living beings. It is the science behind the manifestation of your desires as co- creator based on the power of your ideas, intension and actions. As a co-creator you require purpose, focus and integrity to create a positive, good life.

The Law of Humility; one of the main principles in this law is the quality of having a modest view of one's importance. It includes the mindset of not thinking we are better than other people.

The Law of Growth; this law is based on intentionality, awareness and consistence. Progressive growth, over time helps build a feeling of expectation and desire for the particular thing to happen. Stringing together enough days of consistent growth, is the key to change as a person for the better.

The Law of Responsibility; this law equates to adding conscious thinking before acting. It dictates that you must accept total and complete responsibility for all your decisions, which include what you choose to feel, think, do or say. You become what you think about most of the time. And only you can decide what you think and how you think about it. Therefore, only you are responsible for what happens in you life.

The Law of Connection; this law is based on the principle that everything in life including past, present and future are connected. Who you are today is the result of your previous actions and who you be tomorrow will be the result of your actions today.

The Law of Force; this law states that the time rate of change of the momentum of a body is equal in both magnitude and direction to the force imposed on it.

The Law of Giving; this law states that one must give first before one will receive. According to this law, whatever you give will come back to you in an amazing way. For example; you may give away your time and it comes back to you much later from an unexpected source in an unexpected form in a way that benefits you greatly.

The Law of Here and Now; this law states that to experience peace of mind, one must embrace the present. This is possible, only when you make friends with yourself and let go of negative thoughts or behaviour from the past.

The Law of Change; this law states that everything is in the process of becoming something also. Change is as natural as life, itself.

The Law of Patience and Reward; this law states that we must be consistent in our goals, and they will come to fruition. For example, eating healthy for one day and sabotaging it in the next will not work. Consistency is the key to get good results.

The Law of Significance and Inspiration; this law states that the value of something is the direct result of the energy and intent that is invested in it. Invest your time into something that will be valued instead of blowing your energy on things with no value.

After the expulsion from the Garden of Eden, Adam and Eve had to live together as an imperfect couple estranged from God. Now they were faced with new circumstances dictated by the laws of Cause and Effect. The fall of Adam and Eve is a metaphor that describes the transition of the first man and woman from the state of innocent obedience to God to a state of free will in a world that is ruled by the mixture of the forces of good and evil.

THE LOSS OF INNOCENCE

In Kabbalah, the Tree of Life is not a literal tree but a symbol that is used to explain the nature of God and its relationship to the created world. It is a reflection of man-woman, who are a microcosm of the divine. The Tree of Life and the Tree of the Knowledge of Good and Evil are depicted as a diagram consisting of 10 nodes (Sephirot) symbolising ten different archetypes or dimensions and 22 lines representing 22 energy paths. The Sephirot are arranged into three columns, each defining different aspects of existence, God and the human psyche. And the lines illustrate a web of paths connecting them to one another. The tenth and lowest Sephira represents the Tree of the Knowledge of Good and Evil, Malkut which is regarded as an attribute of God and not a direct emanation from God. Rather it emanates from God's creation, when it reflects and reveals its glory from within itself. Malkut is the dwelling and settling place for the Divine presence known as Shekhinah here on earth. It is considered the presence of God in the form of the Divine feminine energy in the world, and the source of life for the Living Soul (the human being).

By eating of the Tree of the Knowledge of Good and Evil, Eve and Adam linked together heaven and the underworld (death-hell). Their action animated the nebulous presence of evil in the realm of potential, creating an opportunity for evil to mix with good. The mixture of good and evil, took place from the moment they disobey God and ate the forbidden fruit. Their first sin was a "sin of disobedience". Before eating the apple, the concept of evil was foreign, a separate entity from Adam's and Eve's psyche. It was not in their divine nature to crave evil thoughts, speak evil words or perform evil deeds. Eating and absorbing the essence of the forbidden fruit changed all that. They lost their innocence, thus their sex drive and inclination for evil were born.

The Tree of Life which fruit was denied to Adam and Eve depicts the first nine descending nodes "Sephirot", from the Divine consciousness to the material world. When Adam and Eve were first created, the Divine light in them (energy) was pure and they were one with God. After eating the apple, their divinity began to dissipate which led them down the descending worlds of creation to the material world known as the world of Asiyah. As they descended, each lower world became less pure and more dense. And because Adam and Eve did not eat the fruit from the Tree of Life that could have made them immortal, once in the material world, they experienced evil, they suffered, got sick and old until they died. Metaphorically, due to their actions all living beings inherit the same destiny of suffering and in the end death.

The Tree of Life is also called the "Tree of Souls", symbolically, it represents the expanse of the Soul from its highest level "Divine Intellect" to the lowest level "raw sexual energy and survival". It is the downward spiral of the Soul from its original form (the Adam Kadmon or concentration of God's divine light) to the material world. The first four descending Sephirot (nodes) are considered part of the Divine realm. Starting on the fifth Sephira and beyond the physical body began to consume most of the attention of the Living Soul as the Divine light began to disappear. The fifth descending Sephira is closely associated with time, the sixth with space, the seventh with air, the eighth with fire, the ninth with water, and the tenth with earth. The movement and interchange of these elements became the essence of life, here on earth. These elements are essential in the construction of the living being and its senses: smell, taste, sight, touch and hearing. Metaphorically smell is associated with earth, taste with water, sight with fire, touch with air and hearing with space.

The ten Sephirot or nodes in the Tree of Life and Tree of the Knowledge of Good and Evil are connected with 22 lines forming a diagram. This diagram depicts the different dimensions God, the creator used to manifest his Divine light in the process of creating a living universe. And because Eve and Adam, the ultimate accomplishment in God's creation and possessor's of God's Divine light disobeyed and ate the forbidden fruit, they fell from grace. As they descended, each lower dimension they fell into, became more difficult and the Divine light in them less visible. By the time they reached the tenth Sephira or dimension, "Malkut" good and evil were already blended together and God's light appeared to be mostly extinguished.

The ten Sephirot representing the Tree of Life and the Tree of the knowledge of Good and Evil and the seven Chakras, "Shiva's Linga and Shakti's Yoni from the Yoga Tradition are two paradoxical systems. The ten Sephirot show the fall of the Living Soul from the Divine to the Material Realm, and the Chakra system show a way back to the Divine through a process of physical and mental purification. Even though these two system describe two different journeys of the Living Soul, they both consist of pathways that intersect and transport life energy throughout the entire system (the physical body).

In Kabbalah the dwelling place of this life energy (Shekinah) is "Malkut", the Earthly Realm. In Yoga the dwelling place of this life energy (Kundalini) is in the Earth Chakra "Muladhara" at the base of the spine. In both traditions this life energy is considered a feminine energy which animates and gives life to the body, therefore manifesting the "Living Soul" or living human being. Together, the Tree of Life, the Tree of the Knowledge of Good and Evil represent the road map or pathway the Soul took on its way down to the material world. This downward spiral the Living Soul took from the highest realm, the Adam Kadmon (concentration of God's Divine Light) to the material realm manifested four Spiritual Worlds. These four worlds represent the different levels the Soul experienced on its way down the descending chain of Existence. These worlds are synonymous with the four physical realms of human life: spiritual (spirit), emotional (heart), mental (mind), and physical (body).

The Chakra system, is composed of seven vortexes of energy that correspond to specific nerve bundles, glands and internal organs of the body. These Chakras run from the base of the spine to the top of the head. If these energy centres get blocked, they will cause physical and emotional symptoms. The highest of the Chakras (Crown Chakra) is linked to every other Chakra, and therefore to every organ and organ systems of the body. It affects not just those organs, and organ systems but especially the brain and the nervous system. The Crown Chakra is considered the Chakra of enlightenment, it represents the connection to our life's purpose and spirituality.

FOUR SPIRITUAL WORLDS

These "Spiritual Worlds" were animated by the emanations (Sephirot) of the creative life-force from God, the Divine Infinite in the descending chain of Existence, represented by the fall of Adam and Eve (Living Souls). From the beginning, God gave them the gift of choice (free will), which is considered a necessary condition for moral responsibility. And by creating them in his own image God saw them as natural partners in expanding his creation. But partnership requires trust, sadly, the first humans made the choice to trust the serpent over God's wisdom, (historically the snake has been a symbol of fertility, life, healing, transformation and rebirth). And when God confronted them about their decision to eat the forbidden fruit, instead of taking moral responsibility, Adam blamed Eve, and Eve blamed the snake. As punishment for their disobedience, and lack of moral responsibility God banished them from Paradise, and Adam and Eve found themselves tangled up in the descending chain of existence defined by the four Spiritual Worlds. These four worlds consist of the ten Sephirot, each been composed of three Sephirot, except for the last world, the earthy realm which is composed of only one Sephira, Malkut.

Ten Sefirot = Four Spiritual Worlds

First World:
1. Keter - Divine intellect
2. Chokmah - Wisdom
3. Binah - Understanding

Second World:
4. Tipheret - Spirituality & balance
5. Gevurah - Judgement & limitation
6. Chesed - Kindness & love

Third World:
7. Netzah - Eternity & victory
8. Hod - Majesty & splendour
9. Yesod - Foundation upon which God built the world

Fourth World:
10. Malkut - Earth (kingdom)

God began the process of creation by withdrawing his own essence from an area within itself, creating a vacuum where creation could begin. The first emanation in the vacuum (chalal) was in the form of ten "concentric circles" (the Sephirot), after that the Adam Kadmon (Living Soul) emerged in the form of a "man-like" being, covered by the vacuum itself. The Adam Kadmon was the first Divine figure of human likeness (partzuf) to become manifested in the vacuum which resulted from the contraction (tzimzum) of God's Infinite Light (Or Ein Sof). The Adam Kadmon represented pure Divine Light, the highest form of the Soul, possessing no vessel (physical body).

The ten Sephirot defined as ten concentric circles, after Adam and Eve committed the first sin, become the stage for the creation of the four Spiritual Worlds. The energy contained within these circles (Sephirot), the founding element of the Spiritual Worlds was a nebulous, latent potential representing the Supreme essence of mankind and all subsequent descendants, thereafter. In the human psyche the Divine Light of the Adam Kadmon corresponds to the collective and purest essence of the Soul.

"The anthropomorphic name of Adam Kadmon denotes that it contains both the ultimate divine purpose for creation, i.e., mankind, as well as an embodiment of the ten Sephirot. Adam Kadmon preceded the manifestation of the Four Worlds: Atzilut (emanation), Beriah (creation), Yetzirah (formation) and Asiyah (action). In the system of the Sephirot, Adam Kadmon corresponds to Keter (crown), the divine will that motivated creation." - Kabbalah

1. Atziluth (Emanation) is the first Spiritual World, consisting of the first three Sephirot: Kether, Chokomah and Binah. This is the highest level of consciousness, refer to as "Closeness" - Divine Wisdom. This world is eternal, and unchanging, located at the highest level of Tree of life and at the head of the human body. In the human body, it represents the brain, the most important organ of the nervous system. Atziluth is an intellectual world, where ideas, visions and objectives are formalised before been passed down to the lower worlds to be implemented. This world is separated from the other three worlds that form the trunk and roots of the Tree of Life, just like in the human body the brain is separated from the spinal column, torso and extremities. The essence of the world of Atziluth is separated from the divinity and light of God by only one realm.

2. Beriah (Creation - Divine Understanding) is the second Spiritual World, consisting of the following three Sephirot: Tiferet, Gevurah and Hesed. The initial separation of the Living Soul from the Divine light took place in this world. It is located at the trunk of the Tree of Life, and in the human body at the level of the torso, including the spinal column (spinal cord), and the peripheral nervous system originating from the cervical and top thoracic vertebrae the control the arms and hands. Beriah was created ex nihilo (out of nothing) and represents the first true separation from the purely divine. This separation brings several new concepts into play such as; dissimilarity, day, night, past, present, future, male, female, time, imperfection, imbalance change and evil. In this new world the Living-Soul experiences great limitations which lead to feelings of being and self consciousness as opposed to the feeling of "nothingness" experienced in the previous Spiritual Worlds. The throne of God emanated form the light of Beriah world (world of creation).

3. Yetzirah (Formation - Divine Emotions) is the third Spiritual World consisting of the following three Sephirot: Yesod, Hod and Netzah,

located at the lower part of the Tree of Life. In the human body it represents the lower part of the peripheral nervous system, including the pelvic region, legs and especially the penis. After the mixture of good and evil, this world became the abode of the lower angels (sexual desires) of the Living Soul. Biologically, the world of formation starts on the 8th week of fertilisation of the mother to be. At this point in time, the embryo is considered a foetus, named "the formation of the child". During pregnancy, all the parts that have already formed in the womb will grow and develop into a "Living Being" to be born into the material world (Asiyah- earth) where the forces of good and evil are in constant opposition. Once, in this world the child must adopt if he or she is going to survive. Here, the soul (Nefesh) in the child has equal consciousness and awareness of good and evil. The evil side alludes to the feeling of self-awareness and importance (I, me, mine, myself.) and the good side alludes to the genuine desire to help and make others happy.

4. Asiyah (Action - Divine Activity), this is the fourth Spiritual World consisting of the last Sefirah, Malkut. This world represents the Tree of the Knowledge of Good and Evil. In the human body it represents the "Divine Feminine Energy", it is closely associated to the energy of the feminine reproductive system. In this physical world, human consciousness is no longer directly connected to God. Here, human tendencies and identification is with the physical form, needs, wants, pleasure and specially pain. Our identification and dependency of the material world caused the Divine intellect to go dark. The original Living Soul that was projected as the "Adam Kadmon" from the Divine Light as it descended the different Spiritual Worlds became more and more distant from human consciousness and perception. In the material world, the needs of the body became the reality of the Living Soul (Adam Kadmon), placing the Glory of God on the back burner. This is the physical-material world we inherit from our ancestors Adam and Eve due to their disobedience after God told them "Not to eat from the "Tree of the Knowledge of Good and Evil." And to show his disappointment, God cursed Eve with the following words; "I will greatly increase your pains in childbearing; with pain you will give birth to children. Your desire will be for your husband, and he will rule over you". To Adam God said, "Because you listened to your wife and ate from the tree about which I commanded you", "You must not eat, of it," cursed is the ground because of you; through painful toil you will eat, of it all days of your life".

In the material world, human efforts and rituals to communicate with the "God

Head" became for the most part futile. Here, in this realm the Divine Intellect got replaced by the Human Intellect which lead to feelings of self-importance, insecurity, greed, anger, fear and ignorance. The separation from the Light of God, provided independence, intellect and free will but at a great cost and responsibility. It set off the cause and effect process which lead to the "Twelve Laws of Karma".

THE FIVE DESCENDING REALMS OF THE SOUL

1. Yechida, in the human psyche, this realm corresponds to the level of the Adam Kadmon, which illustrates the collective essence and blissful state of the Soul. At this level the Soul is natural, pure and bound to God's original Infinite Light (Ohr Ein Soft). In Yoga this blissful state is known as the "Anandamaya Kosha". The most subtle or spiritual of the five levels of the self.

2. Chaya - This aspect of the Soul sees God in a way that transcends all aspects of existence and physical reality. It corresponds to the World of Atzilut (World of Emanation) and represents the knowledge of absolute truth, considered the essence of life in a state of pure Wisdom. Chaya describes the life Adam had in the Garden of Eden, before eating the forbidden fruit. In this state the Soul is pure, ego does not exist and the communication with God is direct. In Yoga this state is known as "Vijnanamaya Kosha", also known as the Wisdom sheath. This Kosha encompasses intuition and intellect. It is pure awareness, and the first layer of the casual mind located in the Sahasrara, Ajna, and Vishudda Chakras.

3. Neshamah - this aspect of the Soul corresponds to the World of Beriyah (World of Creation). At this level the Soul is endowed with the ability to embrace God's primordial qualities, Wisdom (Chokmah) and Understanding (Binah) representing the conceptual grasp of the intellect. In Yoga, this level is known as "Manomaya Kosha". It is the Mental sheath, composed of manas, meaning "mind." Instinctual consciousness, thoughts and perception are all linked to Manomaya Kosha. This sheath is located in the Heart Chakra (Anahata).

4. Ruach, this aspect of the Soul corresponds to the world of Yetzira (Formation). The primary manifestation of the Soul based on pure Emotional energy. In Yoga this level is called "Pranayama Kosha".

This Kosha is the vital function (breath) or Life Force sheath. Awareness and control of this Kosha allows the Living Soul (person) to move stagnant energy, so he or she can experience greater vitality and energetic connection to the self, others and nature. This sheath is located in Solar Plexus Chakra (Manipura) and Sacral Chakra (Swadhisthana).

5. Nefesh is the lowest aspect of the conscious Soul. It is related to the physical body and the physical world, in the world of Asiya- the world of Action. In Kabbalah, Nefesh is seeing as the awareness of the body. In yoga this level is called "Annamaya Kosha" and it is considered the outermost layer, the gross physical body represented by the flesh, blood, muscles, and bones. The body is nourished and maintain by food so this Kosha is called Annamaya or the food Kosha. This sheath is located in Earth or Root Chakra (Muladhara).

Nefesh is the lowest level of consciousness associated with the physical body and Ruach is the vital breath that animates all living bodies (beings), including animals, alike. In Yoga Ruach is known as "Prana", the essence that animates the living body and the representation of the existence of God in the Material World, the world of Asiyah. Kabbalah states that when a person is born into the lowest and densest form of the Living Soul, Nefesh also called the Tzelem Elokim (meaning the image or reflection of God in the material world), he or she is animated by the power of Ruach. Tzelem Elokim represents the spiritual framework and union of the physical body to the Spiritual Soul. This framework derives from the configuration of the ten Sephirot, which created the four Spiritual Worlds through which the Living Soul descended on its journey into the physical form (body) and the material world.

MASCULINE ENERGY & FEMININE ENERGY

The four Spiritual Worlds represent the Tree of Life and the Tree of the Knowledge of Good and Evil and their association to the different levels of the Living Soul (human being), including physical, mental and spiritual attributes and capabilities. The first nine Sephirot constitute the first three Spiritual Worlds as well as three descending levels of Souls' Consciousness. The fourth Spiritual World represented by the tenth and lowest Sephira, Malkut (Earth- kingdom), is associated with the Divine Feminine Energy known as Shekinah in Kabbalah, and Kundalini Shakti in the Yoga Tradition.

Each Living Soul is a combination of Consciousness associated with masculine energy and the essence of life which is associated with feminine energy. Each and every Living Soul born in the material world is born with both male and female characteristics or energies. When a male "Living Soul" and female "Living Soul" unite into one, via sexual intercourse and "reproduce", the gender of the new Living Soul (child) will depend on the mixing of their sex chromosomes. After nine or so weeks using ultrasound the gender can be revealed. According to science, the child's biological sex "male or female" is determined by the chromosome that the male parent contributes. Boys have XY sex chromosomes while girls have XX sex chromosomes; the father can contribute the X or Y chromosome, while the mother can only contribute one of their X chromosomes.

Boys are endowed with a greater amount of masculine energy which is characterised as assertive, goal-oriented, accomplished and dominant based on logic and reason. Girls are endowed with a greater amount of feminine energy, characterised as nurturance, sensitivity, sweetness, warmth, modesty, humility, empathy, affection, tenderness and kindness. When these energies are balanced within the individual regardless of gender, he or she experience a greater sense of harmony and fulfilment. However the world in general, but specially in the workplace tend to downplay feminine qualities and encourage male characteristics.

According to Kabbalah Shekinah and according to Yoga Kundalini, Shakti are the source of life for all living creatures. Both traditions see this feminine energy as "God's manifested glory" and "God's Divine Presence" in the world. In their respective points of view, these two representations of the same feminine energy is the manifestation of the Godhead as mother, daughter, sister and Holy Spirit. The positive Cabalistic-Yogic perspective of the Divine Feminine energy as God's presence in the material world restores the negative view that was placed upon women by the Judea-Christian culture since their founding.

The purpose of Kabbalah as well as the purpose of Yoga is to cleanse and purify the body-mind system, and bring the feminine energy back to the highest level and reconnect with the Divine Consciousness, Keter (crown) in the Kabbalah Tradition and the Crown Chakra (Sahasrara) in the Yoga Tradition. The return of the feminine energy back to the source of origin will restore the Divinity of the Living Soul. Both traditions present several techniques, including silent prayer and meditation for the stimulation of this feminine energy in order to awaken and begin its ascension up the different Spiritual Worlds or Chakras back to the Divine Intellect.

THE THREE SEFIROTIC PILLARS

The 22 lines that interconnect the emanations of the Tree of Life represent the 22 letters of the Hebrew Alphabet, together with the ten Sephirot form God's 32 paths of mystical Wisdom. These 32 paths represent the different periods in the Divine creative process that manifested the physical universe, including the structure of the human being, called the Tzelem Elokim. Within the Sephirotic structure as well as within the human body three parallel columns are formed: the right column (pillar of Mercy) representing the spiritual force of expansion; the left column (pillar of Severity) representing the spiritual force of contraction; and the middle column (pillar of Awareness) representing balance and union between these opposing forces. In the Tree of Life, the pillars represent different values, electric charges, or types of ceremonial magic. And within the human body, the pillars are associated with the right, middle and left side of the body and functions, mirroring the anatomical Sephirotic structure of the Tree of Life.

Pillar of Awareness: Keter, Tiferet, Yesod & Malkut

1. Keter (Crown-divine intellect) is the second highest realm, just beneath the Adam Kadmon, located at the crown of the Tree of Life. In the human body, Keter is located in the head. It is considered the crown and represents the structure and the functioning brain. This organ is composed of several different parts: The largest part is called the cerebrum and consists of two hemispheres, left and right separated by a bundle of more than 200 million myelinated nerve fibres called the "Corpus Callosum". This bundle of nerve fibres permits communication between the right and left brain hemispheres. Some of the functions the cerebrum emanates are the initiation and coordination of movement and regulation of the temperature in the body. Another major part of the brain is the cerebral cortex, this is the outermost sheet of neural tissue compose of six layers of nerve cells. The cerebral cortex is divided into four lobes as land marks to identify its anatomy and the functions it generates. The neocortex comes next, it comprises the largest part of the cerebral cortex, making up approximately half the volume of the brain. The neocortex is the centre for higher brain functions such as: perception, decision making, language, neuronal computation, attention and memory. Then we have the cerebellum, located at the back of the brain, underlying the occipital and temporal lobes of the cerebral cortex. The cerebellum accounts for approximately 10% of the brain's volume but it accounts for 50 % of the total number of neurones in the brain. This part of the brain helps with coordination and movement related to motor

skills, especially involving the hands and feet. It also helps maintain posture, balance and equilibrium. And deep inside the brain we have the "Limbic system", responsible for behavioural and emotional responses, especially when it comes to actions we need for survival such as, feeding, reproduction, caring for our children, and the fight or flight response. And lastly we have the brain stem, which is a stalklike part of the brain that connects the brain to the spinal cord. The brain stem helps regulate essential functions such as breathing and heart rate.

2. Tiferet (Glory & splendour), even-though is the sixth Sephira of the Tree of Life, it sits right underneath Keter. This emanation stands for balance, beauty, compassion, integration, miracles and spirituality. It represents the spinal column in its entirety, considered the throne of glory and the house of the Living-Soul. Tiferet, stands tall facing East, it has a direct communication with all the other Sephirot and indirect communication with the tenth Sephirah, Malkut. Tiferet is surrounded by Chesed on the right side, facing South, Gevurah on the left side facing North and below Netzach under Chesed, Hod under Gevurah and Yesod directly below Tiferet. Together these six Sephirot become one entity, Zre Anpin, known as the small face of God and the masculine counterpart of Malkut.

3. Yesod (Foundation), the ninth Sephira sits below Tiferet near the base of the Tree of Life and in the human body, it represents the penis. Yesod represents the energy of the male reproductive system and transporter of the seminal fluid into Malkut (Kingdom-womb). This seminal fluid contains spermatozoon (ancient Greek meaning seed or Living Being). Once the seminal fluid is secreted through sexual intercourse into Malkut, one spermatozoon joins an ovum (female reproductive cell) to form a zygote (single cell) with a complete set of chromosomes, that normally develops into an embryo before being born as a living being.

4. Malkut (Kingdom), the tenth and lowest Sephira sits at the bottom of the Tree of Life, just above the world of Qliphoth (Tree of Death). In the human structure, Malkut represents the female physical body, separated from the male physical body. According to Kabbalah, unlike the other Sephirot, Malkut is an attribute of God not a direct emanation. It represents the universal feminine energy and the physical realm of matter, including the earth and female reproductive system. In this material realm the Divine light is hidden and instead of receiving Divine Light, Malkut received life energy becoming the reproductive

mechanism in the material world. The pillar of Awareness reflects the four stages of consciousness: waking consciousness (anything from day-dreaming to intense concentration), preconscious (knowledge and memories), subconscious (below conscious awareness) and unconscious (stores memories you are unaware of...)

Pillar of Mercy: Chokmah - Chesed – Netzah

1. Chokmah (Wisdom), the second Sephira of the Tree of Life sits on the right side of Keter. In the human structure, it represents the right brain hemisphere. The energy from this hemisphere controls the left side of the body via the spinal cord and is responsible for spatial abilities such as attention, vision, imagination, emotions, music awareness, the power to recognise faces and the ability to imply meanings. This Sephira represents the inherent, godly wisdom of the Living-Soul. King Solomon described this wisdom as follows, "For the Lord gives wisdom; from his mouth comes knowledge and understanding. Knowledge and understanding are the tools and wisdom is the craft in which the tools are used".

2. Chesed (Loving kindness), the fourth Sephira of the Tree of Life sits underneath Chokmah. This is an action emanation and in the human structure, it represents the right side of the torso, including the right peripheral nervous system, right arm and hand and the power they represent. In some Kabbalistic circles, Chesed is known as the right hand of God and deals with righteousness, compassion and loving-kindness towards all living beings. Chesed is controlled by Binah, the energy of the left brain hemisphere.

3. Netzah (Eternity), the seventh Sephira of the Tree of Life, located underneath Chesed. It represents the right hip, leg and foot and the power they represent. Netzah, Chesed and Chokmah form the "Pillar of Mercy". This pillar stands for endurance, perpetuity and victory. The principles of long-suffering, strength, endurance and patience are closely held by this pillar.

Pillar of Severity: Binah - Gevurah – Hod

1. Binah (intuitive understanding), the third Sephira of the Tree of Life and sits right across from Chokmah. In the human structure, this Sephira represents the left brain hemisphere which is responsible for controlling the right side of the body. It is credited with the power to understand logical reasoning, comprehension, science, mathematics

and language. While the right side is more dominant in spatial tasks, the left side is more dominant on sequential abilities. In reality, both brain hemisphere with the help of the bundle of nerve fibres that connects them, the Corpus callosum work together to perform both tasks.

2. Gevurah (strength), the fifth Sephira of the Tree of Life sits underneath Binah. It is endowed with emotive attributes and it is consider the great fire of God and giver of The Torah to Moses on Mount Sinai. In the human structure, it represents the power inherited by the left side of the torso, including the left peripheral nervous system, left arm and hand. Gevurah is controlled by Chokmah, the energy emanating from the right brain hemisphere. Benevolence and mercy between people and devotional piety of people towards God and the grace, favour and mercy of God towards people are the virtues of this Sephira. Chesed and Gevurah define God's interaction with the world of opposites, right/left, pull/push, good/evil, pain/pleasure in the material world.

3. Hod (Majesty, splendour, glory), the eighth Sephira of the Tree of Life sits underneath Gevurah. It represents the left hip, leg and foot and the power they represent. Hod, Gevurah and Binah make up the "Pillar of Severity or Pillar of Form". It is the passive, receptive, component in the body containing the Divine Feminine energy. This energy corresponds to mortality, emotions and spirituality.

DA'AT - ANAHATA CHAKRA

The mystical location or state where the ten Sephirot in the Tree of Life are reunited as one is called "Da'at" (Knowledge). In the Yoga Tradition Da'at is represented by the Heart Chakra "Anahata". In Da'at all Sephirot exist in their perfect state, a condition of infinite sharing. This knowledge is hidden behind the veil of ignorance, separating the potential from the actual, a division separating the creator from the created. The location of Da'at is in the region of the heart, described as the void that lies between the three highest Sephirot and everything also that lies below. It is the abstract location of the human soul and life force, similar to the void created by God after contracting the divine light and projecting the image of Adam Kadmon in it. Removing the veil of ignorance, Da'at serves as the connection or bridge to the intellect and the realm of emotions.

Concentrating the ten Sephirot in Da'at through meditation, silent prayer or

yoga, conscious- knowledge and understanding will come about. This mystical experience is regarded as the highest of all the states of consciousness. There is nothing more empowering than the knowledge of Da'at which leads to self-empowering and revelation of the Divine Light known as Shekhinah in Kabbalah or Kundalini-Sakti in the Yoga Tradition. This Presence is manifested in the form of Divine feminine energy, considered the source and mother of all living beings in the "material world". By the power of this Divine energy all living beings in the physical world are animated.
Shekhinah and Kundalini-Shakti are considered the Living Soul and feminine personification of Divine Wisdom residing within all of us.

According to Kabbalah, by the age of three, most children have enough Da'at (knowledge) to start learning the difference between right and wrong. During the adolescence period, Da'at unravels from its cocoon, hormonal changes take place and a new human being unfolds. A state where the "One" is self- knowing, conscious of the realisation that "I am". But it is not until twenty years of age, the sages determined, that most Living Souls develop a "mind of their own". Da'at seems to be closely related to language and improves as the language gets more vast and fluid. The Mishnah "Study by repetition" tells us that one who lacks language and is untrained, deaf and mute has no "Da'at".

JESUS CHRIST - THE SON OF GOD

Jesus' name in Hebrew was "Yeshua", after receiving Sophia (Divine wisdom) in his heart, he became the Christ, the anointed one, the Messiah, son of God. In Christianity, Sophia represents Shekhinah, God's manifested glory and his dwelling place. She is considered, both the creator and the counterpart to Jesus Christ. According to "Gnostic" (meaning esoteric Knowledge) beliefs, Christ was conceived off as having two aspects: a male half, identified as the son of God, and a female half, identified as Sophia, who is venerated as the mother of the universe. Their union is synonymous with the gathering of the ten Sephirot in Da'at where they become "One with God". "Let light shine out of darkness," "made his light shine in our hearts to give us light of knowledge of God's glory displayed in the face of Christ." - 2 Corinthians 4:6
The Christos-Sophia union creates a path back to divinity based on service to others, love of God and respect and obedience of his commandments (Ten Commandments). According to Yogananda, Christ's way was at the heart of his Kriya yoga. He saw the Christos-Sophia path as the way to spiritual awakening, leading back to the Divine Light within one self and within all creation.

According to gnostic beliefs, the Christ-Sophia union represents, "the Sacred marriage of the polarities in creation, including the polarities of gender (male-female) at the spiritual, mental, emotional and material levels". This union of opposing energies is essential for the perception of the Divine Light within the Living Soul in the material realm. Cosmologically, Yogananda explained the Christ-Sophia union as emerging at the beginning of time as the original emanation of the prime creator to fill the empty space with meaning and beauty. Metaphorically, Sophia represents the embodiment of the eternal love and pure feminine radiance and Christ represents, the masculine Divine consciousness, protector of the world and guardian of the Sacred wisdom.

YOGANANDA AND CHRIST

The teachings of Jesus Christ were fundamental in Yogananda's life. Yogananda claimed that his mission, "was to bring the original teachings of Christ and teachings of Krishna (Bhagavad Gita) and show their unity and wisdom to the world". Christ, "The Messiah" as well as Krishna "God of Love" were at the centre of Yogananda's Self Realisation Fellowship Organisation's teachings. Yogananda commented that, Christ was Mahavatar Babaji's guru, and that Christ was the one who asked that his teachings of Self-Realisation in the form of Kriya Yoga be brought to the West.
Mahavatar Babaji was Yogiraj Lahiri Mahasaya's (1828-1895) guru.

Several of Lahiri's disciples, described in several publications and biographies that Babaji appeared to them between 1861 and 1935. And according to Yoganada's autobiography, Babaji has resided for hundreds of years in the remote Himalayan regions of India, seen in person by only a small number of disciples. Babaji's teachings were passed to a long chain of yoga masters that include: Lahiri Mahasaya, Sri Yukteswar Giri, Paramahansa Yogananda, Vishnu Ghosh and Bikram Choudhry, my dear teacher. The continuity of masters that represent this knowledge lives on.

Yogananda knew the Holy Bible very well, he presented the mystical wisdom of the "Old and New Testaments" in his writings and during his lectures. Yogananda held Jesus Christ in the highest of regards and saw many similarities in the teachings of Christ and his own teachings. He even called his personal mission "The Second Coming of Christ." In his Autobiography of a Yogi, Yogananda wrote, "Mahavatar Babaji is in constant communion with Christ; together they send out vibrations of redemption, and have planted the spiritual seeds of salvation for this age." By unifying the wisdom of the Bible with the wisdom of Yoga, Yogananda created a powerful amalgamation of Jewish-Christian-Yogic wisdom. A pathway to understand the nature of the "Soul", leading back to the

"Divine" in a very simple and easy way. If properly understood and applied could revolutionise the world.

TREE OF LIFE - TREE OF YOGA

The Tree of Life based on the ten descending Sephirot describing the fall of the Living Soul from the highest level, the Adam Kadmon (Divine Consciousness) to the earthly, material world known as Malkut (Kingdom). The material world represents the Tree of the Knowledge of Good and Evil and the mixture of righteousness and wickedness, including life and death. In this earthly plane Patanjali, one of the original Siddhars codified the traditional system of eight limbs, known as Ashtanga or Raja (Royal) Yoga, which represents the Tree of Yoga. This Classical Yoga, built on the knowledge of the Vedas and the Tantras lays out a transcendent path, based on eight levels leading back to the Divine state of consciousness. The aim of this Yoga is to teach practitioners how to focus their life energy inwardly in search of the spiritual and permanent truth that lies within each one of us, away from external, sensory, transient world. It is said, that by internalising and concentrating our life energy inwardly the union of the Living Soul with the absolute or the Divine consciousness is not only possible but is our destiny.

PATANJALI - FATHER OF MODERN YOGA

Patanjali, this ancient sage from India is known as the author of the Yoga Sutras and Ashtanga Yoga, also known as Raja or Classical yoga. This Yoga was arranged into a systematic code for practice based on 8 limbs or principles that represent the four classical paths of yoga: Karma Yoga, Hatha Yoga, Bhakti Yoga and Jnana Yoga, which together constitute "Raja Yoga" known as the Royal Path or the Tree of Yoga. The first two limbs: Yama (abstinence) and Niyama (observances) constitute Karma Yoga; Asana (yoga postures) and Pranayama (breath control) constitute Hatha Yoga; Pratyahara (withdrawal of the senses) and Dharana (concentration) constitute Bhakti Yoga and Dhyana (meditation) and Samadhi (absorption) constitute Jnana Yoga. The systematic practice of the 8 Yoga principles or four classical Yogas will lead to a mental state known as Kaivalya, meaning to sharpen one's perception of the self and witness consciousness as a separate entity from matter.
This mental state is synonymous with the Cabalistic sate of the "Adam Kadmon" the body-less Divine light reflected in the void reserved for creation by God.

The human "Living Soul" in the Sutras is referred to as the "Atman", and the highest universal principle as Brahman. Patanjali, in his Sutras states that when avidya (ignorance) is removed from the Atman, human consciousness returns to the Divine Realm and becomes one with Brahman (God), the unchanging Universal Spirit. Brahman is considered "Trimurti" - three Gods in one, with three essential functions required for the universe to exist: Brahma, the source of creation; Vishnu, the preserver of life, balance and harmony; and Shiva, the destroyer of ignorance and evil. Together these three aspects of God create, protect and transform the universe...The Trimurti simply represents three different aspects of the same force.

THE EIGHT BRANCHES OF THE TREE OF YOGA:

1. YAMA

The first branch of the Tree of Yoga is Yama based on five basic "right living or ethical rules" promoting good and ethical conduct presented in the Vedas and the Yoga Sutras. They are a body of moral, imperatives, commandments, and goals leading to mindfulness and a more conscious state of being. According to Patanjali, these rules are essential on the path of Yoga, without them it is almost impossible to form a good Yoga foundation.

The five rules for Right Living are as follow:

1. Ahimsa means nonviolence, is an ancient principle of non-aggression which applies to all living beings. It is a key virtue not only in Yoga but of all Hindu religions such as Hinduism, Buddhism and Jainism as well. Some of the harmful aspects of Ahimsa that need to be avoided or prevented include; asking others to commit violence, encouraging others to commit violence, and assenting, condoning or performing violent acts whether in the physical, mental or verbal form.

2. Satya means truthfulness, this Yama teaches how to think, speak, and act with integrity and truthfulness. Through the practice of Satya we learn how to be truthful with oneself, honest with others, and how to refrain from being judgmental. It presents a way to live life in accordance with the highest standard based on truth, speaking and acting with thought and good intention.

3. Asteya means non-stealing, this Yama is about honesty and respect, not yearning to possess things, especially something that belongs to

others, including their time, peace and experiences.

4. Brahmacharya means moderation, this Yama is based on the practice of "good conduct and moderation" which includes eating a balanced diet, not criticising others, practicing silence for a short while during the day, being conscious about everything we do, not speaking unnecessarily, staying away from bad company, and spending time with nature in the forest or open spaces. Some yogis see Brahmacharya as a reference to a lifestyle defined by sexual continence or complete abstinence.

5. Aparigraha means non-attachment, this Yama states that we must perform our actions to the best of our ability with flexibility and an open mind, without any expectations. Letting go of unnecessary possessions that take up space and energy, in your head as well as in your home is also part of this Yama. Practice self-care, be positive, forgive and be generous.

2. NIYAMA

Niyama is the second branch of the Tree of Yoga. It is also composed on five main observances or disciplines for the purification of the body, mind and soul. These observances are duties and habits for healthy living, and spiritual enlightenment presented in the Vedas and the Yoga Sutras as well. The five observances are as follow:

1. Saucha meaning purity, cleanliness, and clearness of mind is the first Niyama. The first part of this Niyama is based on a group of six physical techniques for the purification of the body called Kriyas: Number one is Dhouti, consisting of a technique to clean the roots of the teeth to prevent dental decay; number two is Basti, consisting on a technique to cleanse of the colon (enemas); number three is Neti, consisting on a technique using water to cleanse the upper respiratory system (neti pot); number four is Trataka, consisting of a meditation technique that involves staring at a single point for extended periods of time; number five is Nauli, consisting of a technique to stimulate the internal organs and cleanse the abdominal region; and number six is Kapalbhati, a breathing technique to strengthen the chest, cleanse the abdominal organs, and energise the circulatory and nervous systems. The second part of the Niyama is creating a clean and pure environment, general personal hygiene, and eating a well-balanced diet

2. Santosha means contentment, and according to Patanjali it refers to the dissolution of desires that block the cultivation of inner peace and

joy. The practice of this Niyama helps elevate the practitioner's state of mind above the day to day challenges and struggles by practicing mindful living, and not wasting energy and time thinking unproductive and wasteful thoughts. The goal is to train the practitioner how to remain calm in success or failure. It is all about creating a positive space in one's mind and in life, so satisfaction, fulfilment and happiness can find a place to live within oneself.

3. Tapas in the Yoga tradition translates as austerities or disciplines for physical and mental purification. The purpose of this practice is to generate physical heat and burn off the impurities in the body to achieve physical and mental health . Some of the best known Tapas include: fasting, abstinence, the practice of Yoga asanas, austerities and penance. They are practiced in order to burn away past karma, and stop producing new karma, for the purpose of achieving Divine consciousness. Tapas are described as the passion to strive to be the very best one can be, based on self study and perfect alignment and coordination with the Divine.

4. Svadhyaya means self study, study of the Vedas and study of other spiritual scriptures. This practice leads to a clearer understanding of the self. It can be done by meditation, spending solitary time in nature and studying wisdom teachings. Gaining a deeper understanding of oneself will help cultivate inner strength and inner peace which are invaluable qualities in difficult situations.

5. Ishvara pranidhana is presented as the one energy expressed through all forms, and thus is often represented as the syllable "OM", as pure vibration.This Niyama represents the spiritual vibrations originating within the human heart. These vibrations can be strengthen by spending time alone, being gentle, practicing gratitude, and finding joy and beauty in everything we do.

The Yamas and Moses "Ten Commandments" which Yogananda embraced as part of his Kriya Yoga reflect a morality essential for "Right Living" in the material or world of Action known as Asiyah in Kabbalah.

3. ASANA

Asana is the third branch of the Tree of Yoga was originally done for the concentration of the mind and for meditation. Patanjali in his Yoga Sutras defined "asana" as a seating position that is steady and comfortable where the student can seat for extended periods of time. The Goraksha Sataka, written in

10th or 11th century and the Hatha Yoga Pradipika written in the 15th century mentioned 84 Asanas, but only a few of them were described. According to these two ancient texts asanas were practiced primarily for physical benefits and mental concentration. Later on, around the 1800's and 1900's, Hatha Yoga incorporated new asanas (body postures) that surpass the 84 number. These new asanas derived from other physical activities such as dance, gymnastics and martial arts which included extension, flexion, balancing, twisting and inverted positions. And in the late 1900s and early 21st Century a new brand of Yoga evolved called "Modern Yoga". The focus of this new way of practicing Yoga became primarily physical with therapeutic benefits. This new Yoga perspective lead to university and independent studies that provided evidence that the practice of asanas improve flexibility, strength and balance; reduce stress and alleviate some chronic illnesses such as arthritis, asthma and diabetes.

4. PRANAYAMA

Pranayama is the fourth branch of the Tree of Yoga. This powerful Yogic practice is done for the purpose of clearing out physical, mental and emotional blockages. Pranayama is generally described as breath control. In Sanskrit "prana" means "life force", which animates the universe, including the human body" and "ayama" means "extension or expansion" of the life force. There are many breathing techniques under this discipline which should be carefully studied before starting their practice. The proper understanding and practice of these breathing techniques will strengthen the lungs and connection between body, mind and emotions. And will soothe and calm the active thinking mind. The first Pranayama exercise is to simply breathe and notice the natural process of the breath. This technique is a necessary step before initiating any of the more difficult Pranayama exercises. The breath is an involuntary and voluntary function in the body that affects the person at every level including the unconscious, emotional, mental and physical.

The combination of asana and pranayama create one of the basic and most important techniques in Hatha Yoga known as "Mudra". It is believed that the practice of Mudras help the connection between the body and mind, soothe pain, stimulate endorphins, improve personal mood and increase vitality.

5. PRATYAHARA

Pratyahara means "gathering towards" or "withdrawal of the senses", it is the fifth branch of the Tree of Yoga. At the root of this practice is the ability to disengage the mind from the constant external disturbances and distractions by withdrawing and concentrating the senses internally. The internalisation of the senses is the beginning of the journey in search of the inner self and awareness of the Soul, the Divine light within our bodies. Transcending the constant sensory stimulation coming from the outside (material world) to the inner self (inner world) will raise the frequencies and vibrations in the body to a higher level of consciousness where the physical, sensual, mental and spiritual energies will merge into one (union of the ten Sephirot in one.) The preferred location in the body for merging these energies is in the region of the heart (heart chakra or Da'at in Kabbalah), therefore reversing and internalising the flow of Prana (life energy) creating a solid foundation for concentration, which will lead meditation and eventually Samadhi.

6. DHARANA

Dharana (concentration) is the sixth branch of the Tree of Yoga. It is a continuation of Pratyahara (withdrawal of the senses), which creates a mind-set where concentration is focused on an object without wavering. Even though the fixing of the mind on a particular object either, externally like on an image of a deity or internally such as on a chakra, internal organ or bodily function are both considered part of Dharana, the internal focus for Self-realisation is far more effective. The objective of the internal focus is to unite the mind, senses and living energy (prana) on a specific place in the body, and quiet the mind which are essential for meditation.

Pratyahara and Dharana constitute Bhakti Yoga, known as Yoga of Devotion and love of the self (Atman) and of God (Brahman). The aim of this practice is "to attain God-realisation", known as "Oneness with the Divine".

7. DHYANA

Dharana is the practice of concentrating the mind on a particular subject and Dhyana is the state in which total concentration has been achieved. At this level of inner focus and awareness, the mind, senses and living energy are united in a specific place within the body, ideally within the region of the heart. This concentration of physical, mental, emotional and energetic forces "into one" transcends the practitioner's attention and awareness to another level of mental clearness and emotional calmness.

8. SAMADHI

Samadhi represents, "total self-collectedness or inner precision", a state of ecstasy, bliss and enlightenment. It is the conscious transcendence and merging of the human Soul with the Divine and highest reality while still attached to the body. Only by a conscious and relaxed focus on the self (Soul) can one achieve this calm-abiding meditative experience.

Dhyana and Samadhi constitute Jnana yoga also known as the Path of Knowledge and Self- realisation. The aim of this yoga is to become liberated from the illusory world of Maya (self limiting thoughts and perceptions) and to achieve the union of the inner self (atman) with the oneness of all life (Brahman) in the Divine Realm.

9. SHIVA'S LINGA - YESOD IN KABBALAH

In the Yoga Sutras, the linga (male genitalia) is considered the purest product of Prakrit (matter). It symbolises the god Shiva and is revered as an emblem of generative power. The health of the "masculine-body" is closely related to the health of his linga. The proper stimulation of the linga generates healing at all levels and for all parts of the body. The linga is one half of the reproductive system, Yoni (female genitalia) been the other half. The Yoni represents the generative power and symbolises the Goddess Shakti. When the Linga and the Yoni come together through sexual intercourse, if both individuals are healthy will lead to pregnancy and eventually form another human being. "The energy of all the chakras is gathered in the linga to be channelled into the Yoni below." - Tantra Yoga

In Kabbalah "Yesod" is the nine Sephira of the Tree of Life and is synonymous with Shiva's Linga. Yesod is considered the foundation upon which God built the world. Yesod also serves as a transmitter between all the other Sephirot above and the reality below. "The light of the upper Sephirot gather in Yesod to be channelled to Malkut below."- Zohar

10. YONI-SHAKTI - MALKUTH IN KABBALAH

Yoni is the symbol representing the goddess Shakti, her feminine generative organs, power and consort of Shiva. In Shivas's temples the linga and the Yogi are often at the centre of his shrines, surrounded by sacred images of deities. It is usually, depicted as a smooth cylindrical mass resting in the centre of a lipped disk shaped object, representing the Yoni. The word "Yoni" has been interpreted as the "womb", "source" and the "female organs of generation", such as vagina, vulva and uterus. The symbol of Shiva and Parvati (Shakti) are represented by the Lingam and the Yoni, symbolising the life force of the universe. It is believed that when they come together, they create a cosmic balance and harmony in nature.

Malkuth is the 10th Sefira in the Cabalistic Tree of Life. Unlike the other nine Sephirot, Malkut is an attribute of God which did not emanated from God directly. It is considered the "Kingdom" and dwelling place of "Shekhinah", the divine feminine energy. This feminine energy can not be seen nor heard, but it can be felt. She is the feminine energy that exists on the earth, including living beings, oceans, moon and trees. Malkut sits at the bottom of the Tree of Life, below Yesod and symbolically, it represents the "Bride" and Tiferet, the sixth

Sephira symbolises the "Bridegroom". These two energies, male-female are the existential dynamic underpinning of all reality according to Kabbalah.

Together, the eight branches of the Tree of Yoga plus the human reproductive systems represented by the Linga and the Yoni are synonymous with the Tree of Life. The different styles of yoga manifested by the limbs of the Tree of Yoga: Karma, Hatha, Bhakti and Jnana Yoga, represent the ascending process the living soul has to travel through each of the Four Descending Spiritual Worlds from Kabbalah that constitute the different dimensions of the Tree of Life. The systematic practice of these yogas lead to the cultivation of self-knowledge, health, discernment, awareness, self-regulation and a higher personal consciousness. Through self-knowledge Yoga shows a way back to the blissful nothingness, the undisturbed, natural state of calm, serenity, peace and communion with the Divine, the Adam Kadmon (Spirit of God.)

YOGANANDA - BISHNU GHOSH & HATHA YOGA

In 1915 Yogananda was initiated into India's ancient swami monastic order by his Guru, Swami Sri Yukteswar. After his initiation Yogananda left his physical practices to devote himself to the spiritual practices of Kriya Yoga therefore passing the baton of physical Yoga (Hatha Yoga) to his younger brother Bishnu Ghosh. As a monk, Yogananda devoted his life time to promote and teach the basic principles for right living and spiritual development based on the first two branches of the Tree of Yoga, the Yamas & Niyamas. These two branches, the Yamas and Niyamas are an essential part on the Royal path of Yoga.

Bishnu Ghosh attended Yogananda's Ranchi School for Boys, where he was trained under the strict supervision of his brother, Yogananda. Bishnu's training consisted on the study and practice of Asanas (yoga poses), Mudras (seals), Bandhas (physical locks), Kriyas (cleansing techniques) and Pranayama (breath control exercises), which are all part of the Hatha Yoga Pradipika Tradition. Later on, after his university education, Bishnu open his own centre of physical education and added weight lifting and muscle control to his curriculum, creating a revolutionary Yoga and Body Culture program. To understand how and why Yoga evolved from very old traditions to the new concepts presented by the Ghosh brothers, pioneers in the development of "Modern Yoga" we must start at the beginning of Yoga, starting with the Siddhars.

THE SAPRISHIS & THE SIDDHARS - THE BEGINNING OF YOGA

The myth- It is said that nearly 15000 years ago, Lord Shiva reached enlightenment and gained super natural powers. Once Shiva reached this blissful state, he started dancing vigorously on top of the Himalayas mountains. His dance is known as "the Ananda Tandava". Shortly there after his performance attracted many people who wanted to learn the secret of his joyful happiness. They gathered around expecting Shiva to come out of his frenzy performance to no avail. After a long while most of the attendants got impatient and left before learning anything about Shiva's blissful state. In the end only seven individuals known as the Saptrishis stayed. They are known as the "mind-born sons"of Brahma, the representation of the Supreme Being as the Creator. The Saptrishis pleaded Lord Shiva to come out of his trance and teach them the secret behind his enlightenment, in vain. After a long time, Shiva finally came out of his trance and told them that in their present state they were not ready to learn from him. He instructed them to practiced sadhana (daily spiritual practice) to prepare themselves for his teachings. They followed his instructions, and faithfully practiced spiritual rituals for 84 years before Shiva finally decided to take them as his disciples.

Shiva as Adiyogi (first yogi) instructed them in the Science of Yoga. After completing their training, shiva commanded them to pass along this knowledge and tradition to all humanity. They got Shiva's blessings and went in different directions to impart the knowledge of yoga and the secrets of enlightenment to anyone who would listen. The Saptarishis are considered the first yoga practitioners on earth.

The number "seven" in relation to the seven Saptarishis was a very important number for the people of the in the Indus Valley or Dravidian Civilisation. This civilisation a "Bronze Age" civilisation was established in the northwestern region of South Asia, lasting from 3300 BCE to 1300 BCE. During the reign of this civilisation, 18 perfected individuals that went by the name of Siddhars dominated the ancient Tamil teachings of philosophy. The myth says that they received the knowledge of the Agamas, "that which has come down" based on cosmology, epistemology, philosophical doctrines, meditation, four kinds of yoga, mantras, temple construction, deity worship and a sixfold system to attained desires from Shiva himself. Patanjali, the compiler of the Yoga Sutras and creator of the Tree of Yoga (Raja Yoga), in the Tamil Siddha Shaiva is considered one of the 18 Siddhars.

The Siddhars were considered saints, known to have had mastered many powers and achieved a "God like state". Based on the writings they left behind and records found in the Harappa region in Punjab and in Mohenjo-daro, near the Indus River, they were skilled in several fields such as: science, astronomy, literature, fine arts, music, drama and dance. Their knowledge about nature and the human body lead them to the creation of the Siddha Medicine and the Varma Kalki, a martial arts system; in my opinion, those are the roots and foundation of "Yoga". The Siddhars were considered the first scientists, saints, alchemists and mystics all in one.

The Varma Kalki is a system of martial arts for self-defence and medical treatment at the same time. The Varman are specific pressure points and pathways located throughout the body, known as "nadis" in the Yoga tradition and "meridians" in Ayurveda and Traditional Chinese Medicine. The nadis, when manipulated can give different results such as disabling an attacker in self-defence or balancing a physical condition as an easy first-aid medical treatment.

The Siddhars discovered that when the "nadis" are blocked, the flow of energy in the body is compromised and illness can happen. To unblock and restore the flow of energy and balance the functions of the body, a series of techniques were developed. These techniques included: diet, herbs, massage, steady poses for meditation and breathing exercises. The Siddhars are known to have being the first to develop a pulse-reading method called "Nadi Paarththal" to identify the origin of different diseases.

FROM SIDDHARS TO SIDDHAS

Three millennia (give or take) later, around the 10th Century AD, another group of ascetics emerged, this time in the Northern part of India and Tibet. This group of ascetics called themselves "Siddhas", instead of Siddhars. The "R" was removed from their name, but not their purpose "to achieve a high degree of physical as well as spiritual perfection". This group of Shivaism monks was lead by Matsyendranath, known as the founder of the "Nath Movement" and creator of Hatha Yoga. The "Naths", meaning lords, protectors and masters adopted Buddhist and Shivaist ideas but more importantly, they refined the ancient Yoga techniques that originated from the Indus Valley Civilisation, codified by the Siddhar Patanjali in his "Yoga Sutras".

This new group of holy men (Siddhas) gave especial attention to the Varma system of nadis (pressure points and energy channels in the human body). And primarily to the Sushumna (spinal cord), pingala (the extroverted, solar nadi, corresponding to the left brain hemisphere), Ida (introverted, lunar nadi, corresponding to the right brain hemisphere) and the set of seven main energy centres align along the spine, the Chakras. The writings of Matsyendranah and

Gorakhnath, the two Siddhas considered the fathers and creators of Hatha Yoga were the principle inspiration for the Hatha Yoga Pradipika (Light on Hatha Yoga.) The techniques in this Yoga manual were the foundation to Vishnu Ghosh's Yogic training.

HATHA YOGA PRADIPIKA

Around the late 14 or early 15 century the Hatha Yoga Pradipika was composed by Swami Svatmarama, a Siddha, himself. His synthesis is based on the work done by Matsyendranath and Gorakhnath, plus other earlier Tantric Practices and Yoga Traditions. It is a guide to the mystic world of Hatha Yoga. In this work, Swami Svatmarana introduced Hatha Yoga as a preparatory stage for the purification of the energy centres and channels (chakras-nadis) in preparation for the higher meditative Yoga practices. The recommended preparatory techniques in his text included: postures (asanas), breath control (pranayama), hand or body gestures (mudras), concentration (dharana), force postures (bandhas) and cleansing techniques (shatkarma also known as Kriyas). Swami Svatmarana stated the the cleansing of the energy centres and energy pathways lead to the purification of all the other bodily systems as well. According to him, without this purification, samadhi or complete absorption with the "Divine" is impossible. All these techniques were at the heart of Bishnu's training based on Yogananda's teachings.

VARMA KALAI MEDICINE

The Varma Kalai is a branch of the Siddha System of Medicine based on vital (pressure) points called Varman. This medicine originated in the Tamil Nadu region in Southern India and is considered the oldest system of medicine, and mother of modern therapeutic disciplines such as Ayurveda, Yoga, Acupuncture, Acupressure and Martial Arts. The main objective of this ancient form of medicine is to balance the biological substances found throughout the human body and mind known as the three Doshas: Vata, Pitta, and Kapha. The meaning of the word Dosha can be translated as "that which can cause problems". These three substances present in the human body and mind are believed to be responsible for the person's physiological, mental, and emotional health. The proper balance of these substances (Doshas) is considered vital for the overall health of the individual.

According to the Varma Kalai philosophy there are over 108 types of Varman (pressure points) that create a network of energy centres and channels in the body.

This network is responsible for the circulation and distribution of all the bodily fluids and pranic, mental and spiritual energies to every organ, tissue and cell in the body. When some of this channels are blocked or poorly functioning, the person can experience circulation problems that often manifest symptoms such as headaches, numbness and tingling in the hands and feet, muscle cramping, fatigue, varicose veins and digestive issues. The most common techniques used in the Varma Kalai system to cleanse this important network of channels and energy centres include massage, alternative medicine, Yoga techniques such as Asana, Pranayama, Mudras, Bandhas and Martial Arts techniques. These practices are done for the purpose of stimulating the body's pressure points (Varman), open the circulatory channels and restore the overall flow of bodily fluids and energy throughout the body.

Varman are also known as "Nadis", they form a network that is closely related to the nervous and circulatory systems. This network of Nadis is responsible for the flow of bodily fluids and energy to all the tissues of the body, including the soft internal organs such as the lungs, heart, and the organs of the digestive, excretory, and reproductive systems. The visceral nervous system, part of the peripheral nervous system relay information between the central nervous system and these internal organs. The nervous system in combination with the blood vessels and other hollow tissues where blood, energy and other substances circulate throughout the body generate the body's vital signs such as body temperature, pulse rate, respiration rate and blood pressure.

The Varma Kali describes the Varman or Nadis as a network of channels, nerves and blood vessels responsible for the distribution of life force (prana) and bodily fluids to the three levels of the human being; the causal body, the physical body, and the subtle body or astral body composed of the mind, ego, and vital energies. In Yogic and Vedantic philosophy the "Causal Body" is the most subtle of the three levels and it is generally referred to as the highest and innermost realm that veils the Atman or true self. The Causal Body is defined as the vehicle for the ego and the seed potential for sensory experiences. According to this philosophy the Nadis originate from the heart region and from the kanda which is synonymous with the root of the reproductive organs located in the pelvic region. The Hatha Yoga Pradipika states that there are 72,000 Nadis which spring out from the three main channels, known as the Sushumna, the Ida and the Pingala. It is said that all the Nadis are connected to the seven Chakras or plexuses along the central channel of the spinal column. And that they are closely associated with the five segments of the spinal column (coccyx, sacrum, lumbar, thoracic and cervical), the pineal gland, the pituitary gland, including the cerebral cortex.

It has been stated that the Sushumna is closely related to the Vagus nerve, the tenth cranial nerve which extends from the brain to the colon with mostly upward firing neurones. The Vagus nerve is also known as the Vagal nerves, which are the main nerves of the parasympathetic nervous system. This system relaxes the body after periods of stress and danger, it also controls specific body functions such as digestion, heart rate and the immune system. The Vagal nerves take a long winding course through the body, reaching from the medulla Oblongata in the lower part of the brainstem down to the neck, chest and abdomen. This nerve is responsible for collecting information from the internal organs, and important glands such as the adrenals, thymus and thyroid, and bring this information to the brain for interpretation.

The Bandhas, a key technique detailed in the Hatha Yoga Pradikipa correlate directly with the path of the Vagus Nerve. This cranial nerve weaves from the brain through the body, carrying information from the body back to the brain. The stimulation of this nerve releases stuck energy in the body, therefore opening the pathway and facilitating the ascent of the Kundalini- Shakti. This ascent takes place in a progressive and systematic way through the different energy centres (Chakras), enabling the practitioner to easily let go of past experiences where he or she may be stuck. This process will lead to grounding spiritual experiences, physical and mental balance and alignment of the conscious mind with the energy of the heart which will reveal the true personality of the Soul.

The Ida Nadi starts at the Root Chakra, Muladhara, runs on the left side of the central Nadi, Sushumna and ends in the left nostril. The Ida Nadi is the introverted, Lunar Nadi corresponding to the right brain hemisphere which controls the left side of the body. This brain hemisphere controls attention, memory, reasoning, and problem solving. When the Ida Nadi is activated, the flow of prana (life energy) to the parasympathetic nervous system known as the rest and digest system is increased, which results in a physical and mental relaxation response. The Ida Nadi has a moonlike nature, represents feminine energy and produces a cooling effect in the body. It is said that this Nadi is responsible for most of the mental and emotional characteristics, and undertakings of the individual.

The Pingala Nadi also starts at the Root Chakra, runs on the right side of the Sushumna, and ends in the right nostril. This Nadi is known for its masculine and heating energy and association with the energy of the Sun. Pingala corresponds to the extroverted processes and to the left brain hemisphere which controls the right side of the body and most of the sympathetic nervous system, which helps the body activate its "fight or flight" response. In general the left brain hemisphere is responsible for language and speech. It has been stated that activating the Pingala Nadi will enhance life processes such as respiration, movement, reproduction, nutrition, growth, and excretion, as well as maintaining the body's vitality, efficiency and strength.

Sushumna Nadi connects the first Muladhara (root) Chakra to the seventh Sahasrara (crown) Chakra, and is the path for the ascent of Kundalini-Shakti up from the base of the spine to the crown of the head. It is considered the central channel for the flow of prana (life energy) throughout the body. Yogis claim that when the Sushumna Nadi is activated and Kundalini-Shakti has been awakened and raised to the top of the head, many psychic powers may develop, such as clairvoyance, telekinesis, telepresence, and even telepathy.

According to the Hatha Yoga Pradikipa, it is essential that Ida and Pingala are properly balanced, before the dormant pathway of Sushumna opens so the goddess Kundalini- Shakti begins her passage up the energy centres (Chakras) towards the Crown Chakra (Sahasrara) known as "the bridge to the cosmos" and final spiritual liberation.

CHAKRAS - NADIS (MERIDIANS)

The Hatha Yoga Pradikipa states that there are 72,000 Nadis, and the Shiva Samhita claims there are 350,000 Nadis running throughout the body. The Nadis are considered pathways of prana (life energy) coextending alongside the visible nervous system and spreading out into finer and finer pathways that reach to every little space in the physical human body. The Chakras and Nadis are part of the same system, the Nadis are considered a boundless network of channels of energy flow found throughout the body, and the Chakras are considered the energy centres and source of this energy flow. The Nadis or Meridians, run on each side of the body, one side mirroring the other.

According to Chinese Medicine there are 12 main Meridians, corresponding to the five Yin-internal organs, six Yang-organs and the Pericardium. The Yin-internal organs include the liver, heart, spleen, lungs, and kidneys. The Yang-internal organs include the gallbladder, small intestines, stomach, large intestine, and bladder. And the Pericardium is a medical concept that describes a set of interrelated parts rather than an anatomical organ. The Pericardium is also called the "heart protector", considered a Yin organ paired with the Yang organ creating the San Jiao or triple energiser.

The Yin and Yang is a Chinese philosophical concept that describes interconnected opposite forces. According to this philosophy, the universe creates itself out of a primary chaos of material energy, organised into Yin and Yang cycles that eventually are formed into living beings. This principle states that all things in the universe exist as inseparable and contradictory opposites, creating pairs of equal opposite forces that attract and complement each other.

These interconnected forces (Yin- Yang) create the vital energy know as Chi, "prana" in the Yoga tradition. Through the practice of different techniques, Chi can be cultivated to promote health, longevity, intelligence, wisdom, and happiness.

YOGA AND THE NERVOUS SYSTEM

The Central nervous system (CNS) is composed of the brain and the spinal cord. It is one of the two parts of the nervous system. The other part is the peripheral nervous system, which consists of nerves that connect the brain and spinal cord to the rest of the body. The CNS can be broken down into several parts: the cerebral hemispheres, the mid brain, the cerebellum, the diencephalon, the pons, the brain stem, the medulla oblongata, and the spinal cord. In terms of tissue, the CNS is divided into grey matter and white matter. The grey matter comprises neurones (nerve cells), axon terminals, and dendrites, as well as all nerve synapses. Most synapses are chemical, and communicate using chemical messengers. Other synapses are electrical, in these synapses, ions flow directly between cells. Grey matter is abundant in the cerebellum, cerebrum, and brain stem. White matter is found in the deeper tissues of the brain. It contains nerve fibres (axons), which are extensions of the nerve cells (neurones).

Each part of the CNS plays an important role in how the body functions, together all of these parts take in information and control how the body responds. The brain controls most of the functions of the body, including awareness, movement, thinking, speech, and the five senses of seeing, hearing, feeling, tasting and smell. The spinal cord carries messages back and forth between the brain and the nerves that run throughout the body.

The autonomic nervous system is part of the peripheral nervous system. It regulates involuntary physiological processes including heart rate, blood pressure, respiration, digestion, and sexual arousal. This system is made up of two antagonistic sets of nerves the sympathetic and the parasympathetic, plus the enteric nervous system. Together they form a mesh-like system of neurones that control all the internal functions and physical movements of the body. The Enteric nervous system controls the functions of the gastrointestinal tract.

The hypothalamus is a gland located right above the brainstem, considered the body's control centre. It receives autonomic regulatory input from the limbic system (a group of structures deep in the brain which are associated with functions such as memory, emotion, and fear) to keep the body in a stable state called homeostasis. This amazing gland coordinates and controls the body's hormonal system by releasing hormones to the pituitary gland, which sends them out to all the internal organs. By linking the nervous system and the endocrine system by way of the pituitary gland, the hypothalamus regulates many functions of the Autonomic nervous system.

The Autonomic nervous system is a control system that works for the most part autonomously, without one's conscious effort. The two main parts of the Autonomic nervous system, the Parasympathetic and Sympathetic nervous systems originate from two different locations of the central nervous system; the parasympathetic nerves originate in the neurones and cells located in the brainstem and the sympathetic nerves arise from the spinal cord. The sympathetic nervous system goes into action to prepare the body for physical and mental activity. The Parasympathetic nervous system causes a general slowdown in the body's functions in order to conserve energy.

There is a theory that the autonomic nervous system depends on the network of Nadis (channels) for the circulation of life energy covering the entire body. A healthy autonomic nervous system produces and distributes an abundance of vitality, energy and keeps the body young. The parasympathetic nervous system is responsible for the body's rest, digestion, relaxation, resting, or eating. It basically undoes the body's quick involuntary response to danger or stressful situations the sympathetic nervous system produces.

The sympathetic and the parasympathetic nervous systems are controlled by respiration. When one nostril is dominant, the contra lateral brain hemisphere is active. For example, when the right nostril, controlled by the left side of the brain is open and breathing takes place through it, leads to increased sympathetic activity. And when the left nostril is open and breathing takes place through it decreases the sympathetic activity and increases the parasympathetic tone. In Yoga terms; the left nostril is connected to the Ida network of Nadis controlled by the right brain hemisphere and the right nostril is connected to the Pingala network of Nadis controlled by the left brain hemisphere; and when both nostrils flow together, the main channel, Sushumna is stimulated and awakened.

SYMPATHETIC NERVES

The nerves of the sympathetic nervous system, form the sympathetic chain or trunk, usually composed of 21 or 22 pairs of nerves: 3 in the cervical region (neck), 10 or 11 in the thoracic region (upper spine), 4 in the lumbar region (lower spine), 4 in the sacral region (sacrum area) and a single nerve lying in front of the coccyx (tail bone) called the ganglion impair. These nerves (sympathetic nervous system) prepare the body for physical and mental activity.

They make the heart beat stronger, opens airways so breathing is easier, etc. The sympathetic nervous system is triggered by the hypothalamus after receiving a distress signal from the amygdala. The distress signal is sent via the autonomic nerves to the adrenal glands which respond by pumping adrenaline hormones into the bloodstream. The autonomic nervous system has a direct role in the physical response to stress as well.

Another function of the hypothalamus is to connect the nervous system to the endocrine system via the pituitary gland. It controls the hormones released by the endocrine system and sends them to the cells throughout the body. These hormones control mood, growth, organ functions, development, metabolism and reproduction. Together, the autonomic nervous system composed of the parasympathetic nerves, sympathetic nerves, and the limbic nerves plus hormones from the endocrine glands create the different plexuses in the body. In yoga, these nerves and plexuses are considered the channels (Nadis) and energy centres (Chakras). The Chakras are described as spinning wheels and centres where life energy, feelings, emotions and thoughts are converged.

PARASYMPATHETIC NERVES

The main four cranial nerves belonging to the parasympathetic nervous system are the oculomotor, facial, glossopharyngeal and vagus. The parasympathetic nervous system indirectly affects the nerves belonging to the five senses. The longest parasympathetic nerve is the vagus nerve, this nerve contains both, sensory and motor fibres. It originates in the medulla oblongata part of the brain stem, it runs down into the neck, enters the thorax and crosses the left side of the arch of the aorta (the main artery that carries blood away from the heart to the rest of the body) and descends behind the root of the left lung, forming the posterior pulmonary plexus. This plexus is bordered by the superior edge of the pulmonary artery and the lower edge of the pulmonary vein. It contains somatic and visceral afferent and efferent neurones; afferent neurones carry nerve impulses to the brain and spinal cord and efferent neurones are motor nerves, carrying neural impulses away from the central nervous system, toward the muscles to generate movement.

The parasympathetic and sympathetic nervous systems are two halves of the same whole, work at the same time, often in opposition to one another. These two systems are essential for regulating many vital functions, including respiration and the ability of the heart muscle to contract. These functions are controlled and managed by the hypothalamus, located just above the brain stem. The hypothalamus acts as an integrator for autonomic functions, receiving autonomic regulatory inputs from the limbic system. The limbic system is the part of the brain that deals with emotions and memory.

Another function of the hypothalamus is to connect the nervous system to the endocrine system via the pituitary gland. The hypothalamus also controls the hormones released and send by the endocrine system to the cells in the body which control mood, growth, organ functions, development, metabolism and reproduction. Together, the different parts that comprises the autonomic Nervous System: parasympathetic, sympathetic, enteric and limbic nerves plus hormones from the endocrine glands form the seven main body plexuses or Chakras in the human body. Two of these Chakras are located in the head and controlled by the parasympathetic nervous system and the other five are located within the five spinal segments belonging to the sympathetic nervous system:

The practice of Yoga, including Pranayama (breath control) and meditation have been proven to improve the function of the Autonomic nervous system by decreasing the sympathetic, fight or flight response and increasing the parasympathetic, rest and digest tone. The calming effect generated by the practice of Yoga has been shown to generate positive benefits such as improving digestion, strengthening the function of the immune system, reducing hypertension, asthma, and stress-induced psychological disorders.

PARASYMPATHETIC CHAKRAS:
1. Head (pituitary gland) - Crown - Sahasrara Chakra
2. Pineal Gland - Third Eye - Ajna Chakra

SYMPATHETIC CHAKRAS:
3. Cervical Plexus - Throat - Vishuddha Chakra
4. Cardiac & Pulmonary Plexuses - Heart - Anahata Chakra
5. Enteric (gastrointestinal) Plexus - Solar Plexus - Manipura Chakra
6. Lumbar Plexus - Sacrum - Svadhisthana Chakra
7. Pelvic Plexus - Coccyx - Muladhara Chakra

PARASYMPATHETIC CHAKRAS:
1. Sahasrara - Crown Chakra
The Crown chakra is closely associated with the pituitary gland and the hypothalamus together they regulate the endocrine system. This chakra is connected to the higher brain (Divine intellect) and the Supreme Self. The opening and blooming of the this chakra, known as the thousand-petalled lotus represent the complete unfolding of consciousness. The divinity of this chakra is Shiva in the form of pure, Supreme consciousness. The natural element associated with the Crown Chakra is "thought".

2. Ajna - Third Eye Chakra

The third eye chakra is located in a part of the brain which can be made more powerful through concentration and meditation. This chakra is linked to the light sensitive, pineal gland. It produces melatonin, the hormone which regulates the instincts of going to sleep and awakening. Perception, awareness and spiritual communication depend on this chakra and related tissues. It also allows contemplation, self reflection and visionary perspectives. And it helps determine one's reality and beliefs based on what we choose to see in the world. It is the chakra of perception and discrimination. The natural element ruling this chakra is "light".

SYMPATHETIC CHAKRAS:
3. Vishuddha - Throat Chakra

The throat chakra is closely associated with the thyroid and parathyroid glands and the brachial plexus which determines the nature and quality of our nervous system. The nerves that form the branchial plexus are the lower four cervical nerves and the first thoracic nerve (C5, C6, C7, C8 and T1). This plexus is part of the purification centre, that allows the nectar of immortality (Amrita) to drip down from the Bindu chakra located between the crown chakra and the third eye chakra.

Vishuddha chakra is associated with higher discrimination and self-expression. The Hatha Yoga Pradikipa claims that meditation upon this chakra brings forth occult powers such as: "control of the three periods of time past, present and future; freedom from disease and slows down the ageing process; protection from any danger and the ability to control the three worlds: heaven, earth and the underworld". The natural element ruling this chakra is "space". It provides us with the space and freedom to move and express ourselves at will.

4. Anahata - Heart & Lungs Chakra

The heart & lungs chakra is closely associated with the thymus gland and the cardiac & pulmonary plexuses. The cardiac plexus receives impulses from the vagus nerve and the sympathetic trunk of nerves. It controls heart rate, cardiac out put and the contraction forces of the heart. The nerves from the cardiac plexus originate from both the sympathetic and parasympathetic nervous systems. The sympathetic nervous system releases "norepinephrine" a hormone which accelerates the heart rate and the parasympathetic nervous system releases "acetylcholine" a hormone which slow down the heart rate. And the pulmonary plexus is an autonomic plexus formed from pulmonary branches of the vagus nerve and the sympathetic trunk. This plexus is a continuation of the deep cardiac plexus.

The energy represented by this chakra is associated with the element of "air".

The heart chakra serves as a bridge between the lower and the upper chakras.

5. Manipura - Gastrointestinal Chakra

The gastrointestinal chakra is closely associated with the pancreas, the outer adrenal glands, the enteric nervous system and a large division of the peripheral nervous system which controls the gastrointestinal functions. The gastrointestinal system depends on several different types of neurones for it to function efficiently. For example, the neurones within the wall of the bowel control the ability of the organism to move independently, using metabolic energy (motility), blood flow, uptake of nutrients, secretion, and the inflammatory processes in the gastrointestinal track.

The Manipura chakra spins in the area around the abdomen above the belly button up to the breast bone. It represents the source of personal power, self-esteem, warrior energy and the power of transformation. Blockages in this chakra can be related to diet and are often experienced through digestive issues like ulcers, heartburn, eating disorders and other digestive problems. The energy represented by this chakra is associated with the element of "fire". It is directly linked to the sense of self.

6. Svadhisthana - Sacral Chakra

The sacral chakra is closely associated with the adrenal, testicles and ovary glands and the lumbar plexus. This chakra represents the network of nerves that supplies impulses to the skin and the muscular frame of the legs. It is formed by the lower thoracic and lumbar vertebral nerve roots (T12 to L5) which supply motor and sensory innervation to the lower limbs and the pelvic girdle. This chakra is closely associated with creativity and awareness. The energy represented by this chakra is associated with element of "water". It is the place where fear is conquered.

7. Muladhara - Pelvic Plexus Chakra

The Muladhara or Root chakra is closely associated with the Adrenal Cortex glands and the pelvic plexus. These glands produce the hormones that control sex (androgens, oestrogen), salt balance in the body (aldosterone), and sugar balance (cortisol). It is the singular site in the autonomic nervous system where sympathetic and parasympathetic neurones originate from the same nerves. These neurones control the organs involved in elimination of waste from the body and its reproductive functions. The Root Chakra is located at the base of the spine, when heathy, it reproduces a grounding, safe and secure feeling. In this chakra the most basic, instinctual instincts of survival are initiated. The Muladhara is associated with the "earth" element.

The Chakra system and the Nadis are part of the same network; the Chakras are the epicentres and origins of energy (prana) and the Nadis are the infinite network of tubular organs and channels throughout the body where this energy flows to reach and sustain every cell in the body. The purification of the body, Chakras and Nadis is essential for the proper flow of energy and create a perfect physical and mental balance. The three main bodily functions to eliminate waste products from the body are respiration, defecation and urination. The balanced functioning of the systems, responsible for these cleansing functions of the body depend on the health of the energy centres (Chakras) and the network of channels (Nadis) that connects them.

In Yoga, Pranayama or breath control is associated with the purification of the energy centres, pathways and blood to maintain "prana" living energy strong and healthy. "When breath is inhaled, oxygen from the air comes in contact with the impure blood and the blood takes oxygen. The waste matter in the blood releases carbonic acid and the blood is purified."

Defecation and urination are the other two essential functions for the elimination of bodily waste. Poor removal of this waste causes pollution and toxicity which lead to major health problems. The mechanism that generates these bodily functions depends on the communication between the parasympathetic nerves and Nadis controlled by the right side of the brain and the enteric nervous system. Maintaining balance in the intestinal microbial community and intestinal health also depends on this communication. Urination or release of urine is also controlled by parasympathetic nerves and Nadis that trigger the bladder to contract. We urinate to flush out waste products from the body. It also keeps body's fluid levels down, when this fails to happen, "we get fluid build-up in the form of oedema - commonly seen in the form of puffy ankles."

LIVING SOUL - HUMAN ORGANISM

The human body is a complex network of cells that in unity create tissues, organs, passages (ducts) and eventually organ systems. In combination, all of these systems create a magnificent machine that functions and moves, with the ability to perform many different physical and mental tasks efficiently and even reproduce other living beings. The human body can be divided into nine different parts: the head, neck, chest, abdomen, pelvis, back, hips, extremities, and trunk. The relationship and proper alignment between the body's anatomical parts are crucial during the practice of Yoga.

CELLS

The are over 200 different cell categories in the human body. Each category specialising in specific functions. Each particular function performed by the cell, either solely, but usually by forming tissues are essential for the survival of the organism. The tissues formed by the cells grow by increasing the number of cells that make them up. Cells in many tissues in the body divide and grow very fast until the individual reaches adulthood. Once an adult many cells in the body mature and become specialised on their particular function. The tissues formed by the cells, make up the internal organs, which function like factories where every cell has its own specific job. Specific organ groups join together to form organ systems, in which they work in conjunction to carry out specific functions to keep our organism running. Our amazing, human body is composed of all the components of life, organised into different levels such as: chemical, cellular, tissues, organs, and organ systems which together form the human organism.

Some of the most important cells include:
> Stem cells: embryonic and adult stem cell
> Red blood cells
> White blood cells
> Platelets
> Nerve cells: neurones, neuroglia cells
> Muscle cells: skeletal, cardiac, smooth
> Cartilage cells
> Bone cells: osteoblasts, osteoclasts, osteocytes, lining cells
> Skin cells
> Endothelial cells - lining body cells
> Epithelial cells - lining body cavities
> Fat cells: white adipocytes, brown adipocytes
> Sex cells: spermatozoa, ova.

TISSUES

There are four basic types of tissue in the human body, each designed for specific functions:

1. **Connective tissue**; this tissue connects, supports, binds, or separates other tissues or organs, normally having relatively few cells embedded in an amorphous matrix, often with collagen or other fibres, including cartilaginous, fatty, and elastic tissues.

2. **Epithelial tissue**; this tissue forms the outer covering of the skin and also lines the body's cavities. It forms the lining of the respiratory, digestive, reproductive and excretory tracts. This tissue performs various functions such as absorption, protection, sensation and secretion.

3. **Muscle tissue**; this tissue is made up of cells with special abilities to shorten or contract in order to produce physical movement. There are three types of muscle tissue: skeletal muscle attached to bones which allows movement; smooth muscle located in many internal organs; and cardiac muscle, specific to the heart.

4. **Nervous tissue**; this tissue is found in the brain, spinal cord, and nerves. It is responsible for coordinating and controlling most of the body's activities. It triggers muscle contraction, produces environmental awareness, and plays an important role in memory, reasoning, and emotions.

ORGANS

There are 78 organs that make up the human organism, together they give rise to the different organ systems in the human body. From these 78 organs, five of them are considered vital to the survival of the body: brain, liver, lungs, heart, and kidneys. From all the organs that constitute the human organism, the skin is considered the largest one of all, covering the entire body. It makes up about 16 percent of the body's mass, and protects it from environmental stressors like germs, pollution, and radiation from the sun. The skin also regulates body temperature, receives sensory information, and stores water, fat, and vitamin D, to be used when the body needs it.

Brain

An adult, healthy human brain has an average of 86 billion neurones, and 85 billion non-neuronal cells, with 100 trillion connections, which send signals throughout the body. The average weight of this amazing organ is about 1.36 kilograms, its size is about two clenched fists. The brain is divided into two halves, which are connected by the corpus callosum, a large bundle of more than 200 million myelinated nerve fibres, permitting communication between the right and left sides of the brain. The right hemisphere controls the muscles of the left side of the body, and the left hemisphere controls the muscles on the right side of the body. In general the left hemisphere controls speech, comprehension, arithmetic, and writing. The right hemisphere controls creativity, spatial abilities, artistic and musical skills. Overall, the brain processes information, interprets sensation, and controls behaviour and regulates how we think and feel.

Liver

The liver is the largest solid organ in the human body, weighing approximately 3-3.5 kilograms. It is located beneath the rib cage and lungs, in the upper right area of the abdomen. This dark reddish- brown organ consists of two main lobes, each lobe is made-up of four segments, together the two main lobes comprise an average of 1000 lobules. These lobules are connected too small ducts (tubes) that connect with larger ducts, eventually forming the hepatic duct, the tube that carries bile from the liver. At any given time, the liver holds about one pint (13%) of the body's blood supply.

Over 500 vital functions have been identified with the liver including the regulation of most chemicals in the blood. The liver is responsible for the production of bile (consisting of waste products, cholesterol and bile salts) that is secreted by the liver cells to perform two primary functions: to carry waste away, and to break down fats during digestion. It is responsible for the production of proteins for blood plasma, cholesterol and especially proteins to help carry fats throughout the body. It turns excess glucose into glycogen for storage (glycogen can be converted back to glucose for energy when the body needs it). It regulates the levels of animo acids in the blood, which form the building blocks of proteins. It process haemoglobin for use of its iron content. It clears the blood off drugs and other poisonous substances. It regulates blood clotting, plus many more amazing functions are credited to the liver….

Lungs

The lungs are a pair of spongy, air-filled organs located on either side of the chest. The trachea (wind pipe) conducts inhaled air into the lungs through its tubular branches, called bronchi (part of the airways). The bronchi, divide into smaller and smaller branches (bronchioles), finally becoming microscopic. The bronchi move the air to and from the lungs, keeps the air moist, and screen out unwanted particles. The lungs contain all the components of the bronchial tree beyond the primary bronchi. Bronchi is the plural form for bronchus. The left bronchus delivers air to the left lung, and vice versa. On average an adult healthy male can roughly hold 6 litres of air in his lungs. During respiration, the lungs warm the air to match the body's temperature and moisturises it to the humidity level the body needs. At the cellular level, the oxygen contained in the air one breathes is exchanged for a waste gas called carbon dioxide. The bloodstream then picks up and carries this waste gas back to the lungs were it is removed from the bloodstream and then exhale (breathe out), before taking another inhalation. This gas exchange is essential to life.

Heart

The heart is the main organ of the circulatory system, about the size of two hands clasped together. It is located in the front and middle of the chest, behind and slightly to the left of the sternum (breastbone). The heart runs on the power of the brain and the nervous system, and consists of four muscular chambers: two upper atria and two lower ventricles which are powered by electrical impulses. The right atrium receives the oxygen-poor blood from the body and pumps it to the lower right ventricle, in turn the lower right ventricle pumps the oxygen-poor blood to the lungs to be oxygenated and delivered to the upper left atrium. The left atrium receives the oxygen-rich blood from the lungs and pumps it to the lower left ventricle which connects nearly all organ systems in the body through its pumping function. The oxygen-rich blood is circulated through the arteries, which are responsible for the distribution of hormones, and other vital substances in the body. The veins are responsible to bring the deoxygenated blood and other metabolic waste back to the heart to continue this detoxification process. The heart is also responsible for maintaining blood pressure.

Kidneys

Most people have two kidneys, each one about 10-15 cms long, roughly the size of a small fist. The kidneys are located at the bottom of the ribcage, one on each side of the spine. People can live a healthy life with only one functioning kidney, although some complications may develop over time. Each kidney contains about 1 million filtering units, responsible for removing toxins from the blood and transforming waste products into urine. Each kidney weights about 160 grams and gets rid of between one and one and a half litter of urine per day. The two kidneys together can filter up to 200 litres of fluid every 24 hours. When the kidneys malfunction, harmful toxins and excess fluid will build up in the body, which may cause kidneys failure. That is why it is of upmost importance to stay hydrated. Drinking the right amount of water on the daily basis will help the kidneys stay healthy by removing waste products from the blood in the form of urine. The right amount of water will also help keep the blood vessels open so the blood can travel freely to the kidneys, and deliver essential nutrients to them.

Bladder

The bladder is a muscular organ. Located in the pelvic cavity. It stretches to store the urine produced by the kidneys and contracts to release it.

Stomach

The stomach is a muscular, elastic, pear-shaped bag, located crosswise in the abdominal cavity beneath the diaphragm. Its main function is digestion of food through production of gastric juices which break down, mix, and turn the food into liquid.

Intestines

The intestines are located between the stomach and the anus and are divided into two major sections: the small intestine and the large intestine. The function of the small intestine is to absorb most ingested food. The large intestine is responsible for absorption of water and excretion of solid waste material.

Pancreas

The pancreas is located behind the stomach. It is a vital part of the digestive system, and responsible for regulating blood sugar levels.

Spleen

The spleen controls the level of white cells, red cells and platelets. It filters the blood and removes any old or damage red cells from the blood.

Gallbladder

The gallbladder stores bile produced by the liver and then releases it when necessary.

There are many more organs of great importance in the human body. They are special tissues that function in a particular manner. These tissues are connected and constructed as constituents to serve a common function. All organs of the human body work in sync to form about a dozen organ systems. Below is a list of all the organs of both, male and female human bodies, in semi- alphabetical order: Adrenal glands, anus, appendix, bladder (urinary), bones, bone marrow, brain, bronchi, diaphragm (muscle of breathing), ears, oesophagus (food pipe), eyes, fallopian tubes, gallbladder, genitals, heart, hypothalamus, joints, kidneys, large intestine, larynx, liver, lungs, lymph nodes, mammary glands, mesentery (covering of the intestines), mouth, nasal cavity, nose, ovaries, pancreas, pineal gland, parathyroid glands, pharynx, pituitary gland, prostate, rectum, salivary glands, skeletal muscles, skin, small intestine, spinal cord, spleen, stomach, teeth, thymus gland, thyroid, trachea, tongue, ureters, urethra, uterus, skeleton, ligaments, tendons, blood cells, vagina, hair, vestibular system of the ear, placenta, testes, nails, vas deferens, seminal vesicles, bulbourethral or Cowper's glands, penis, scrotum, parathyroid glands, thoracic ducts, arteries, veins, capillaries, lymphatic vessels, tonsils, nerves, subcutaneous tissue, olfactory epithelium (nose), cerebellum.

EXOCRINE DUCT GLANDS - ENDOCRINE DUCTLESS GLANDS

In anatomy a duct is described as a channel or vessel from an exocrine gland or organ through which fluid is distributed to specific regions of the body. The common cardinal veins, also known as the ducts of Cuvier, are a pair of large venous veins that conduct blood to the sinus venous during prenatal development. Arteries and veins are blood vessels containing only smooth muscle cells which form the channels where blood flows through in the body. Arteries carry blood rich in oxygen away from the heart to the different tissues throughout the body. Each artery is a muscular tube made up of three layers: the adventitia (connective tissue anchoring the arteries to nearby tissues), the tunica media (a layer of muscle that lets arteries handle the high pressures from the heart), and the intima (the inner layer lined by smooth tissue called endothelium). And the veins collect and push oxygen poor blood back to the heart. Veins can be categorised into four main types: pulmonary, systemic, superficial and deep veins. Pulmonary veins carry oxygenated blood from the lungs to the heart. Systemic veins are arranged into three groups: 1. Veins of the heart. 2. Veins of the upper extremities, head, neck, and thorax, which end in the superior vena cava. 3. Veins of the lower extremities, abdomen, and pelvis, which end in the inferior vena cava. Systemic veins transport blood from the body tissues to the right atrium of the heart.

The stomach primary or main ducts arise from the stomach wall, which is covered with ciliated cells, composed of microscopic projections that look like tiny hairs, while secondary ones are non- ciliated secretory epithelial cells that contribute to the mucous lining of the intrapulmonary airways. The liver ducts is a network of small tubes that carry bile inside the liver, called the intra-hepatic bile network. This network passes through and drains bile from the liver. The smallest ducts are called ductules, they come together to form the right and left hepatic ducts, which lead out of the liver. The left hepatic duct drains bile from the left half of the liver and joins the right hepatic duct which end up forming the common hepatic duct. The common hepatic duct carries bile from the liver and gallbladder, through the pancreas, and into the small intestine.

Exocrine glands have ducts that carry their secretory fluids to the surface of the skin. These glands include the sweat, sebaceous and mammary glands. Sweat glands consist of two types: eccrine and apocrine. Eccrine glands are found all over the body and open directly onto the surface of the skin. Apocrine glands open into the hair follicle, leading to the surface of the skin. The sebaceous glands are microcosmic exocrine glands that open into the hair follicles to secrete an oily or waxy matter, called sebum, which lubricates the hair and the skin. The mammary glands is a highly evolved and specialised system found in each breast. This system consist of 10-20 simple glands responsible for producing and secreting milk, which is taken though the lactiferous duct, made of about 10 channels in each breast to the nipple.

ENDOCRINE DUCTLESS GLANDS
The major glands of the endocrine system are hypothalamus, pituitary, thyroid, parathyroid, pineal, thymus, pancreas, ovaries, testes, adrenal. These glands

are ductless glands which comprise of feedback loops of hormones released by them directly into the circulatory system. The pituitary gland is called the "master gland" because it controls the functions of all the other glands in the body. The glands in the endocrine system secrete hormones that help cells communicate with each other. They are responsible for most every cell, organ, and function in the body. The hypothalamus, pituitary and pineal glands are in the brain. The thyroid and parathyroid glands are in the neck. The thymus is in between the lungs, the adrenals are on top of the kidneys, the pancreas is behind the stomach, the ovaries (female) and testes (male) are in the pelvic region.

Even though the glands produce very small amounts of hormones, they play an important role controlling and regulating many bodily functions. Hormones control heart rate, sleep cycles, sexual function, and reproduction. Metabolism, appetite, growth and development, mood, stress, and body temperature are all affected by hormones. Overall, hormones play a big role on how one feels, both mentally and physically.

ORGAN SYSTEMS AND FUNCTIONS:

1. Skeletal System
The skeletal system supports the body, gives shape, allows movement, produces blood cells, protects the internal organs and stores minerals. This system has 270 bones, give or take and reaches maximum density around age 21. The bones in this system are connected to one another forming three different types of joints: fibrous (immovable), cartilaginous (partially movable) and synovial (freely movable). Around the joints are strong elastic tissue called "ligaments" that connect bone to bone, give support and limit their mobility. The best known ligaments, because of their exposure to injury are the ones in the knees, ankles, elbows and shoulders. Over stretching or tearing a ligament can cause pain and instability in the joint. Level 1 and level 2 tears, with the proper treatment will recover within three to eight weeks. Parts of this treatment should include resting, wearing a knee brace and doing physical therapy. However, if the ligament is fully torn, you may need to have surgery to repair it.

2. Muscular System
The muscular system, together with the skeletal system form the "musculoskeletal" system which supports and produces the body movements. The musculoskeletal system allows physical movement, maintain posture and circulate blood throughout the body. It is an organ system composed of skeletal, cardiac and smooth muscles. Each type of muscle having its unique compositions and a specific

function: skeletal muscles move bones and other tissue, cardiac muscles contracts the heart and pump blood and smooth muscles located in the walls of hollow organs, arteries and veins contract and push food and blood forward.

Skeletal muscles are attached to bones with tough bands of fibrous connective tissue called tendons. This connective tissue stretches over the joints, contribute to their stability, mobility and can withstand great amounts of tension. Tendons are found throughout the body, from the head to the feet. The Achilles' tendon in the ankle and the tendons in the knee and rotator cuff in the shoulder are of great importance for the stability of the body. When in good shape, tendons improve posture and body movements. Tendons are very strong but prone to injury if the body is not properly aligned. Resistance and weight bearing exercise (standing yoga poses) can strengthen the tendons and ligaments in the legs, pelvic region, abdomen and back.

One of the most important skeletal muscle in the body is the respiratory muscle called the diaphragm, located underneath the lungs. This is a large, dome-shaped muscle separating the thoracic and abdominal cavities. Upon inhalation, the diaphragm contracts and flattens causing the chest cavity to expand. This contraction creates a vacuum, which pulls air into the lungs. Upon exhalation, the diaphragm relaxes and returns to its dome like shape and air is forced out of the lungs. Diaphragmatic contractions are rhythmically and continually and most of the time involuntary. For deep breathing, the diaphragm requires assistance from other muscles, including muscles in the abdomen, the back and the neck. The proper training and development of the diaphragm and the other respiratory muscles came into focus early on in the development of Hatha Yoga. This part of Hatha Yoga is known as pranayama, the practice of breath regulation for physical and mental wellness. The word "pranayama" is composed of two Sanskrit words: "prana" meaning life energy and "yama" meaning control.

Torso
The torso includes: the thorax, the abdomen and the perineum. The most important organs are located within the torso. In the upper chest, the heart and the lungs are protected by the rib cage and the rib cage is protected by the muscles covering it. The abdominal area does not have a bony frame, like the chest does, but it has several layers of muscles that protect the digestive organs housed in the abdominal cavity.

During the third stage of the process of swallowing (oesophageal) the stomach receives the food and mixes it with a watery, colourless fluid known as the gastric acid to help break down the food in the process of digestion. This helps the body absorb the nutrients easier as the food moves through the digestive system. Respectively, the liver produces bile, a digestive fluid which is stored in the gallbladder. Bile helps break down fats into fatty acids, which can be taken into the body by the digestive tract. In the lower part of the alimentary canal we find the small and large intestines which extract the nutrients from the food.

The small intestine helps further digest food coming from the stomach, it absorbs nutrients (vitamins, minerals, carbohydrates, fats & protein) and water from the digested food so they can be used in the body. The large intestine is a long tube like organ that is connected to the small intestine at one end and to the anus at the other. Partly digested food moves through the cecum into the colon, where water, nutrients and electrolytes are removed. By the time food mixed with the digestive juices reaches the large intestine, most digestion and absorption has already taken place. Then there is the anus, the opening where the gastrointestinal tract ends and exits the body. The anus start at the bottom of the rectum, the last portion of the colon (large intestine) and ends at the circular muscles called the external sphincter ani externus. This is a ring-shape muscle that relaxes or tightens to open or close a passage or opening in the body.

The muscles attached to the torso, spine and rib cage form a shield to protect the internal organs by covering them and absorbing shock and reducing friction in the joints. The muscular system is essential in maintaining normal body temperature. As much as 85% of the body's heat is generated by muscular contractions.

3. Reproductive System

The human reproductive system is located in the pelvic region, the lowest part of the torso. This system includes, both the male reproductive system which functions to produce and deposit sperm; and the female reproductive system which functions to produce egg cells, and protect and nourish the foetus until birth. The female reproductive system includes the ovaries, the fallopian tubes, the uterus, the cervix, and the vagina. In men, it includes the prostate, the testes, and the penis. This system is also known as the genital system responsible for four basic functions: to produce egg and sperm cells; to transport and sustain these cells; to nurture the developing offspring; and to produce hormones.

4. Somatosensory system - Skin - Touch

The somatosensory system is composed of somatic senses that respond to touch or tactile perception. This system is a complex network of sensory neurones and natural pathways that help humans recognise objects, discriminate textures, generate sensory-motor feedback and exchange social signals. It is believed that the somatosensory system begins in the receptors located in the skin, joints, ligaments, muscle, and fascia. The receptors that detect changes in the environment are called exteroceptive receptors located in the skin, and the receptors that detect changes within the body are called the proprioceptive receptors. The somatosensory system is endowed with the ability to interpret the sensations of the body, including touch, pressure, vibration, temperature, itch, tickle, and pain. The receptors in the skin and inside the body translate this sensory information and sends it to the spinal cord before reaching the brain.

Upper extremities - arms

In the human anatomy, the arm extends from the shoulder joint to the elbow joint and the forearm extends from the elbow joint to the hand. The forearm is made up of the ulna and radius bones.

These two long bones form a rotational joint, allowing the forearm to turn so that the palm of the hand faces up or down. The muscles of the arm include muscles attach to the scapula, the thorax, and the humerus (arm bone). These muscles are responsible for the movements of the arm, forearm, wrist and hand.

Hand - dexterity

The major function of the hand in all vertebrates except humans is locomotion. The human hand is a miracle in the evolutionary process. Our elongated thumb opposes our four fingers which help manipulate objects and instruments with great precision. The function of the human hand evolved from being a locomotion instrument into a gripping, grasping instrument with the ability to form precise movements. The hand is made up of the wrist joint, the carpal, metacarpal and phalange bones. The thumb is considered a digit, but not technically a finger, although many people don't make a distinction between the thumb and the other digits. All the movements of the arm and hand depend on muscular contraction.

Lower extremities - locomotion

The lower extremity (leg) includes the hip, upper leg, knee, lower leg, foot and toes. In human anatomy, the upper leg is called the thigh and the leg is considered between the knee and the ankle joint. The tibia (shin bone) is the medial bone of the leg and is larger than the fibula, which it is paired with. The tibia, is the main weight-bearing bone of the lower leg and the second longest bone of the body, after the femur. The muscles of the lower extremity are many and complex, including: psoas major and minor, gluteus, lateral rotators, thigh, calf and foot muscles. All the standing poses depend on the shin bone and foot for support and on the leg muscles for their practice. These poses are considered weight baring exercises which can help develop bone density in the legs, hip joints and lower back.

The heart
The heart is an organ-muscle the size of one's fist that pumps blood throughout the body. This organ-muscle has four chambers, two atria and two ventricles... The right ventricle pumps blood carrying carbon dioxide to the lungs so one can exhale it out. The left atrium receives oxygen rich blood from the lungs and pumps it to the left ventricle. The left ventricle pumps the oxygen rich blood throughout the body. This cycle happens for as long as we are alive. At the moment of death the heart stops.

The rhythm and rate of a beating heart is controlled by the parasympathetic nervous system. The lungs are part of the respiratory system and their main function is to move fresh air into the body while removing waste gases from the body. The heart, blood vessels and the blood makes up the cardiovascular system, responsible for three main functions: maintain blood flow, transport nutrients, oxygen and hormones to the cells throughout the body and the removal of metabolic waste products from the body. This is the process that keeps the person healthy and alive. Any malfunction of this process causes toxicity in the body creating an imbalance that will lead to illness or worse.

5. Circulatory System

The circulatory system consists of three independent systems that work together: the heart (cardiovascular), lungs (pulmonary), and arteries, veins, coronal and portal vessels (systemic). The circulatory system delivers oxygen, nutrients and hormones to all the tissues of the body and removes carbon dioxide and other waste products from the body. The heart is a pump, usually beating about 60 to 100 times per minute, during respiration its beating sends blood throughout the body, carrying oxygen to every cell. After delivering the oxygen, the blood returns to the heart, then it circulates back into the lungs to pick up more oxygen. This process repeats over and over again for as long the person is alive. The circulatory system is made up of blood vessels: arteries and veins that carry blood away from and towards the heart. The arteries carry blood rich in oxygen away from the heart and veins carry blood load it with carbon dioxide back to the heart. The arteries and veins travel in one direction only, to keep things running smoothly.

6. Respiratory System

The respiratory system is a network of organs and tissues responsible for the breathing process. It helps the body absorb oxygen from the air we breathe so our internal organs can function. This system consists of airways, lungs, blood vessels and the muscles that power the lungs during respiration. All of these tissues work together to move oxygen throughout the body and remove waste gases like carbon dioxide from the body. The rate and depth of breathing is automatically controlled, unless you are practicing deep or controlled breathing.

The respiratory centres that controlled breathing, receive information from the peripheral and central chemoreceptors and closely monitor the partial pressures of carbon dioxide and oxygen in the arterial blood. Oxygen is essential for every function the body executes to stay alive, this includes digesting the food we eat, moving the muscles during physical activity or even just thinking requires oxygen. These bodily functions produce carbon dioxide which is then removed and exchanged for oxygen by the lungs. In Yoga to increase the exchange of gases in the body Pranayama was developed. Pranayama is a Sanskrit word meaning extension of the breath or more accurately, "extension of life". Proper rhythmic, slow and deep breathing, strengthens the respiratory system, soothes the nervous system and improves concentration.

7. Digestive System

The digestive system consisting of the gastrointestinal tract plus other digestive organs that breakdown the food we eat into smaller and smaller components, until they can be absorbed and assimilated into the body. Once the food is broken down into nutrients, the body uses it for energy, growth and cell repair. Digestion works by moving food through the gastrointestinal (GI) tract. The smooth muscles in the gastrointestinal tract control digestion by moving the food with a wave-like motion called peristalsis. The muscles in the digestive organs contract and relax to cause this movement, which pushes food through the oesophagus into the stomach.

The upper muscles in the stomach relax to allow food to enter, while the lower muscles mix the food particles with stomach acid and enzymes. Then the digested food moves from the stomach into the intestines by peristalsis from there the waste product eventually exit the body through the rectum and anus as feces. To keep the digestive system working well, Hatha yoga techniques such as balanced diet, fasting, yoga poses, body mudras (poses with special breathing), and kriyas also known as shatkarma (cleansing and purifying internal-physical and mental techniques) were developed.

8. Lymphatic System

The lymphatic system is part of both, the circulatory and immune systems. It consists of a network of tissues, vessels and organs that work together to move a colourless, watery fluid called lymph back into the blood stream which consists mainly of plasma. In adult bodies, some 20 litters of plasma flow through their arteries, smaller arteriole, vessels and capillaries. Plasma is the largest part of the blood, constituting 55% of the total blood in the body. No organ produces plasma, instead it is formed from water, salts and enzymes absorbed through the digestive system. The main role plasma plays is to distribute nutrients, hormones and proteins to the parts of the body that need it. Cells dispose of their waste products into plasma as well.

Universally, plasma is called the "fourth state of matter" and comprises over 99% of the visible matter. In the universe plasma is superheated matter - so hot that the electrons are ripped away from the atoms forming an ionised gas. The other three states of matter are: solid, liquid and gas.

The major parts of the lymphatic system are located in the bone marrow, spleen, thymus gland, lymph nodes and the tonsils. This system has several functions including: protecting the body from illness-causing invaders, absorbing digestive tract fats and removing cellular waste. It's vessels drain into collecting ducts, which empty their contents into the two subclavian veins, located under the collar bones. These veins join to form the superior vena cava, the large vein that drains blood from the upper body into the heart. In yoga you will find many different techniques to improve the flow of lymph and remove toxins from the body. Some of these techniques include: alternating yoga poses, staying hydrated, breathing exercises and a healthy diet.

9. Nervous System

The nervous system is a highly complex part of the human body that coordinates its functions and transmits signals between its different body parts. In humans the nervous system consists of two main parts, the central nervous system (CNS) and the peripheral nervous system (PNS). The CNS contains the brain and the spinal cord which are responsible for controlling, regulating and communicating all the functions within the body, including all mental activity such as though, learning and memory. The PNS consists of the nerves and ganglia outside the brain and spinal cord. This system is responsible for sending information from the different body parts back to the brain, as well as carrying out commands from the brain to the different parts of the body. Together with the endocrine system, the nervous system regulates and maintains homeostasis which is the condition of optimal functioning for the organism, including temperature and fluid balance. One of the principal objectives in yoga is to maintain the state of homeostasis in good working condition by improving and balancing the internal, physical and chemical components responsible for maintaining the living organism, healthy.

10. Endocrine System

The endocrine system is made up of organs called glands which produce and release hormones that target specific cells in the body. This system is controlled by the hypothalamus, located on the undersurface of the brain, just below the thalamus and the pituitary gland to which is attached by a stalk. The endocrine system is a chemical system that produces and secretes hormones directly into the circulatory system to distribute and regulate cell activity throughout the body. Hormones are the body's chemical messengers that carry information and instructions from one set of cells to another. The endocrine system consists of:

1. Hypothalamus
2. Pituitary
3. Pineal
4. Thyroid
5. Parathyroid
6. Thymus
7. Adrenals
8. Pancreas
9. Ovaries
10. Testes

The hypothalamus, pituitary and pineal glands are located in the brain, the thyroid and parathyroid in throat, the thymus in the chest right behind the sternum, between the lungs, the adrenals on top of the kidneys, the pancreas behind the stomach in the upper part of the abdomen, the ovaries on either side of the uterus in women and the testes located inside the scrotum in men. Collectively all the glands in the body produce around 50 different types of hormones that control nearly all the processes in the body. These chemicals help coordinate the body's functions from metabolism to growth including, reproduction, sleep, heart rate, appetite, mood, sexual health and even sleep.

Out of the 50 different hormones that have been identified in humans, 14 are described on the listed below:

1. Adrenocorticotrophic hormone (ACTH), this hormone is produced and secreted by the anterior pituitary gland. Its main function is to

regulate cortisol (stress hormone) which is released by the adrenal glands. ACTH also regulates blood pressure, blood sugar, the immune system, and the response to stress.

2. Luteinising hormone (LH), this hormone is made by the pituitary gland as well, and plays an important role in sexual development and function. In women, LH helps control their menstrual cycle, and triggers the release of eggs from the ovaries.

3. Follicle-stimulating hormone (FSH), this hormone in women helps control their menstrual cycle and stimulates the growth of eggs in the ovaries. The level of FSH change throughout the menstrual cycle, with the highest levels taking place just before an egg is released by the ovary.

4. Prolactin (PRL), stimulates breast development and milk production.

5. Melanocyte-stimulating hormone(MSH), describes a group of hormones produced by the pituitary gland, hypothalamus and the skin cells. These group of hormones is important to protect the skin from UV rays, development of pigmentation and controls appetite.

6. Thyroid-stimulating hormone (TSH), this hormone controls the production of the thyroid hormone. When the thyroid hormone levels in the blood are too low, the pituitary gland makes more TSH to tell the thyroid gland to work harder. When the thyroid levels are too high, the pituitary gland makes less or no TSH.

7. Growth hormone (GH), this hormone is secreted by the anterior lobe of the pituitary gland. It stimulates the growth of bodily tissues, including that of the bones.

8. Oestrogen is a sex hormone responsible for the development and regulation of the female reproductive system and sex characteristics.

9. Progesterone is a sex hormone involved in the menstrual cycle, pregnancy, and embryogenesis in women, and gets their uterus ready for pregnancy.

10. Testosterone is the primary sex hormone in males. It plays a key role in the development of the male reproductive tissues, such as testes and prostate, as well as enhancing bone mass, muscles and hair growth.

11. Insulin is made by the islet cells in the pancreas. This hormone controls the amount of sugar in the blood by moving it into the cells, where it can be used by the body for energy. Insulin helps regulate blood sugar levels.

12. Cortisol (stress hormone) is made by the adrenal glands. This hormone affects almost every organ and tissue in the body. It plays several important roles, including: regulating the body's stress response, helping control the body's use of fats, protein and carbohydrates, and plays and important role on the body's overall metabolism.

13. Adrenaline is produced by the adrenal glands and by a small group of neurones in the medulla oblongata. Adrenaline makes the heart beat faster and the lungs breathe better and more efficiently.
It causes the blood vessels to send more blood to the brain and muscles, increases blood pressure, makes the brain more alert, and raises sugar levels in the blood to produce more energy.

14. Melatonin, this hormone is produced by the pineal gland in the brain at night, and is released in response to darkness. It has long associated with control of the sleep-wake cycle. Melatonin provides a circadian and seasonal signal to the organism.

Yoga developed several practices, which include diet, yoga mudras, breathing exercises, relaxing and meditation to stimulate the endocrine system. The aim of these yogic exercises is to harmonise and balance hormonal levels in the body for optimal health.

11. Immune System

The immune system is a network of cells and proteins that defend the body against infection. This amazing system keeps record of every germ or microbe it has defeated so it can recognise and destroy it quickly if it enters the body again. Bone marrow and the thymus gland are the primary organs of the immune system. They produce special white cells called lymphocytes which help the body fight off infection. The lymph nodes, the spleen, the tonsils and certain tissue in the mucous membranes of the body are the secondary organs of the immune system.

The human body has three types of immunity:

1. Innate immunity - every one is born with this immunity, it is a natural immunity.

2. Adaptive immunity - this immunity develops throughout our lives, when we are exposed to diseases or when we are immunised against them with vaccines.

3. Passive immunity - this immunity is borrowed from another source and it lasts a short time. For example, antibodies in mother's breast milk give babies temporary immunity to diseases the mother has been exposed to.

12. Lymphatic System

The immune system is a complex collection of cells and organs that destroy or neutralise pathogens that would otherwise cause disease or death. And the lymphatic system is the network of vessels, cells and organs that carry the lymph (extracellular fluid) to the bloodstream and filters pathogens from the blood. The lymphatic system is a part of the immune system, it produces and releases white blood cells (lymphocytes) and other immune cells to monitor and then destroy foreign invaders, such as bacteria, viruses, parasites and fungi, that may enter the body.

Research has shown that the practice of yoga is a helpful way to boost the immune system and reduce inflammation in the body. For example, breathing exercises contribute to a strong lymphatic system by removing waste gases such as carbon dioxide and other impurities from the body. In addition the contraction and relaxation of the muscles during the practice of yoga poses act as a pump for the lymphatic system. The poses help pump lymph from stagnant areas in the body back into the lymphatic vessels and bloodstream helping detox the body. The right subclavian vein plays an important role in this process.

13. Integumentary System

The integumentary system is the group of organs that consist the outermost layer of the human body. It comprises the skin and its appendages (hair, nails and exocrine glands), together they form the physical barrier between the external environment and the internal part of the body. The primary function of this system is to protect the inside of the body from dangerous elements in the environment such as: bacteria, pollution, and UV rays from the sun that may otherwise cause harm. This system also retains fluids, eliminate waste products and regulate the body's temperature.

14. Urinary System

The urinary system, it also known as the renal system or urinary tract, consists of: kidneys, ureters, bladder, urethra, prostate, renal pelvis, penis or vagina. This system is responsible for the elimination of waste from the body, regulation of blood volume and blood pressure, control of electrolytes and metabolites and regulation of blood pH. The kidneys produce the urine and accounts for the other functions of the urinary system. The ureters carry the urine away from the kidneys to the urinary bladder, which is a temporary reservoir for the urine. When is time to urinate, the brain signals the bladder muscles to tighten, squeezing urine out of the bladder. At the same time, the brain signals the sphincter muscles to relax. As the muscles relax, the urine exits the bladder through the urethra. This system depends on both smooth and skeletal muscles and together with the nervous system work to hold and release urine from the bladder. For normal urination to occur, all the signals must take place in the correct order.

Sensual organs and their functions

The human body has five basic sensual organs: eyes (sight), ears (hearing), nose (smell), mouth (taste) and skin (touch), they connect us to the world around us. These organs contain receptors that relay information through sensory neurones to the appropriate places within the nervous system. With information gathered by the senses, one can learn and make more informed decisions. For example, a bitter taste, can alert us to potential harmful food. Sensations are collected by the sensory organs and interpreted in the brain. This is done by a specialised brach of the nervous system called the sensory nervous system. It is responsible for gathering and sending the constant flood of information from the environment to the brain. The brain depends on colour, shape, and feel of the objects nearby to determine what they are.

Eyes - sight

The eyes collect light from the visible world and convert it into nerve impulses to the brain, which forms an image of the given object. Each eye depends on six skeletal muscles to control its movements. These muscles work quickly and precisely to allow and maintain a stable image, scan the surrounding areas and track moving objects. Any damage to the eye muscles can compromise vision. Some of the techniques Hatha yoga developed to strengthen the eye muscles included "trataka" a purification technique that involves staring at a single point for extended periods of time. The Hatha Yoga Pradikipa defines "trataka" as "looking intently with an unwavering gaze at a small point until tears are shed".

Ears - hearing

The primary function of the ear is to maintain our sense of balance and hearing.

The ear is divided into three parts: the external, middle and inner ear. These three parts are attached but work separately to do their job. The cochlea, a hollow, spiral-shaped bone works with the parts of the outer and middle ear to help make the sounds audible. Specialised receptors called hair cells in the inner ear are responsible for hearing and balance. These receptors change the movement of the fluid within the ear into electrical impulses that are transmitted to the hearing (auditory) nerve, and up the brain, where they are interpreted as sound. The tensor tympani and the stapedius muscles contract to protect the inner ear in response to loud noise. When activated, these muscles reduce the amount of sound levels in the middle ear by dampening vibrations of the ossicular chain. The inner ear also called labyrinth of the ear helps with equilibrium and orientation in space. Balance postures, mantras and other concentration exercises were created in Yoga to strengthen and balance the fluid movement in the ears.

Nose - smell

The nose serves as the entrance to the respiratory tract and contains the olfactory organs. It provides air for respiration, serves the sense of smell, conditions the air by filtering, warming and moistening it, and cleans itself of foreign debris extracted from inhalation. The cells and neurones in the nose capture odours and send signals to the smell centre at the base of the brain, known as the olfactory bulb. The upper respiratory tract, consisting of the nose, nasal cavity, pharynx and larynx allows us to breath and speak. The nose is supported by bone at the back of the bridge and by cartilage in the front and high in the nose are a large number of nerve cells that detect odours. In order to smell, the inhaled air must be pulled all the way up to reach and come in contact with the odour nerve cells. Smell and taste are closely connected. Pranayama was developed based on the nose and its functions.

Mouth - taste

The two main functions of the mouth are eating and speaking. The trigeminal nerve provides sensation (feeling) and helps us bite, chew and swallow. Within the mouth the salivary glands produce and secrete the extracellular fluid known as saliva. It is mostly made of water but it also contains substances essential for digestion. There are over 50 pairs of muscles in the mouth that work together to make chewing, swallowing and talking possible. Inside the mouth we find the most obvious muscle the tongue, it consists of eight interwoven muscles covered in receptors known as taste buds. The tongue also plays an important role in holding the chewed food within the mouth before it transports it to the pharynx. In yoga smiling is considered an exercise. Just breathe in and smile - the tension will disappear and you will feel better. And the yogi diet is based on the principles of purity, nonviolence and balanced living.

Throat - swallowing

The muscles in the throat are responsible for making the complex process of swallowing possible. Some 50 pairs of muscles and many nerves work together to receive food into the mouth, preparer it and move it from the mouth to the stomach. This process happens in three stages: oral, pharyngeal and oesophageal. The oral phase is the voluntary movement of the bolus (food) from the mouth into the oropharynx. The tongue plays an important role in this process by pushing the food to the back of the mouth towards the pharynx, the muscles in the throat contract to push the food down. The pharyngeal phase depends on the involuntary movement of the food from the oropharynx into the oesophagus. And the third phase, also an involuntary movement pushes the food through the oesophagus into the stomach. The swallowing reflex is mediated by the swallowing centre in the medulla (the lower part of the brain stem), which causes the food to be moved back into the pharynx and the oesophagus by rhythmic and involuntary contractions of several muscle in the back of the mouth, pharynx and oesophagus. During swallowing, the larynx muscle contracts tightly to halt breathing and allow food to pass safely. In Yoga the throat is the location for the fifth chakra - Vishuddha. This chakra is the gateway for energy between the lower parts of the body and the head, guided by principles of expression and communication.

Vertebral column (spine)

The spine is regarded as one of the most important parts of the body. It provides structure, support and without it standing up wouldn't be possible. It is made up of 33 vertebrae (bones) stacked up on top of one another forming a strong pillar. Each vertebra has two sets of facet joints, one pair facing upward and the other facing downward which gives certain regions of the spine great range of motion. In between the vertebrae there are 23 shock-absorbing discs, known as spinal discs or intervertebral discs. They are in between the vertebrae acting as cushions, or shock absorbers for the spine. The vertebrae are covered with tendons, ligaments, muscles and other tissues reaching from the base of the skull to the tail bone. The spinal cord and the fluid surrounding it are housed within the spine and together with the brain, form the central nervous system.

The spine provides the body's base support that allows standing, bending and twisting safely and effectively. The human spine is divided into four different regions: the cervical (neck), thoracic (upper back), lumbar (lower back), sacral (pelvic) and coaxial region. The cervical section is made up of the top seven vertebrae (C1-C7), and is connected to the base of the skull. The top two vertebrae are known as the atlas and the axis, which form the joint connecting the skull to the spine. The cervical section is responsible for mobility and normal functioning of the neck, as well as protection of the spinal cord, arteries and nerves that travel from the brain to the body.

The thoracic section of the spine is located at the chest level, between the cervical and the lumbar vertebrae (T1 to T12) and serve as attachments to the ribs. The lumbar section is located between the thoracic vertebrae and the sacrum ((L1 to L5). They are the main weight-bearing section of the spinal column. The sacrum is the section located at the base of the spine. It does not have discs separating the vertebrae, because its five vertebrae (S1 to S5) are fused together. The pelvis is connected to the spinal column at the sacrum section. The coccyx is at the very base of the spinal column and is made up of four vertebrae that are fused together as well.

The spine have some normal, gradual curves when view from the side. The neck and lumbar sections of the spine have a nordic curve, which means that they curve inward. The thoracic spine have a kyphotic curve, which means that it curves outward. These spinal curves help maintain balance while upright and support the weight of the head and upper body. However, too much curvature may cause spinal imbalances, worsening spinal conditions that may result in pain and loss of mobility. A normal adult spine is positioned over the pelvis, so upright posture doesn't strain the muscles. However, changes of the spinal position can stress muscles and cause spinal deformity. If the spine is injured and unable to function properly, it can be very painful or even disabling.

The central focus in Yoga is the spinal column. Consciously practicing Yoga poses helps decompress the spine providing a feeling of space. Medically, decompression of the spine is a non- surgical procedure intended to relieve pressure on the spinal cord or compressed nerve roots passing through or exiting the spinal cord. Spinal decompression therapy aims to help patients who suffer from debilitating pain due to bulging, degenerating or herniated discs.

SPINAL CORD

The spinal cord is a long, thin, tubular bundle of nerve tissue that extends from the base of the brain to the level of the first or second lumbar vertebrae. This column of nerves passes through a hole in the centre (spinal canal) off each vertebra. It extends lengthwise along the back in the spinal canal, giving off pairs of spinal nerves that carry the impulses to and from the brain. The spinal nerves carry electrical signals from the brain to the skeletal muscles and internal organs via the spinal cord. Similarly, they carry sensory information like touch, pressure, cold, warmth, pain and other sensations from the skin, muscles, joints and internal organs to the brain via the spinal cord. All Yoga traditions believe that the energy of the spinal cord is a form of the Divine feminine energy that animates and gives life to the body. Yoga refers to this divine energy as Kundalini Shakti, and in Kabbalah is known as Shekhinah, identified as the daughter of God. One of the principle objectives in Yoga is to liberate this energy and let it flow freely through the seven energy centres (Chakras) to reach an expanded state of consciousness. And in Kabbalah the principle objective is for this energy to return to the divine state by uniting the ten Sephirot of the Tree of Life in the region of the human heart, called Da'at.

Kundalini Shakti

Kundalini-Shakti has several symbolic representations from a coiled serpent at the base of the spine to the natural intelligence of the embodied consciousness in every human being. In sexuality, Kundalini-Shakti is the reproductive energy associated with the manifestation of new living beings. It is also credited as the source of all the feelings of pleasure and pain humans experience in the daily basis. For as long this "coiled power" in reference to a "dormant serpent" in the Muladhara or Earth chakra at the base of the spine remains dormant, will keep the person in darkness and ignorance. It is said that when awaken this energy becomes synonymous with the Supreme Mother Goddess (Devi Durga), representation of the feminine aspect of the power of Brahman, the Supreme God force present within all things.

The ultimate aim in the practice of Yoga is to awaken this coiled power by directing Prana (breath, life-energy) into the Sushumna Nadi, which runs down the central axis of the body through the spinal cord. This Nadi (channel) connects the seven Chakras, from the first Muladhara to the seventh Sahasrara at the top of the head creating a pathway for the Kundalini-Shakti to ascend. Upon awakening, this energy moves upwardly through the Sushumna, unblocking the seven energy centres (Chakras) that roughly correlate with the five spinal plexuses (coccygeal, sacral, lumbar, branchial, cervical), the pineal gland and pituitary gland. The pituitary gland and the hypothalamus work together to regulate the endocrine system responsible for the body's biological processes. In essence, Kundalini awakening is the process of improving circulation and reviving dormant areas of the central nervous system (brain & spinal cord) which result in self-awareness and spiritual enlightenment. When fully awaken, Kundalini-Shakti engulfs the body, mind and senses with Divine energy generating a sense of spiritual bliss, freedom and union with the Divine consciousness (moksha).

Yogananda once said; "The yogi reverses the searchlights of intelligence, mind and life force inward through a secret astral passage, the coiled way of Kundalini in the coccygeal plexus, upward through the sacral, the lumbar, and the higher dorsal, cervical, and medullary plexuses, and the spiritual eye at the point between the eyebrows, to reveal the Soul's presence in the highest centre (Sahasrara) in the brain".

The Cabalistic Shekinah (dwelling or vehicle) represents the same principle as Kundalini-Shakti, and when awaken it is said to follow the mystical path of the Tree of Life back to the Divine. This path is represented by the realms or emanations of the ten Sephirot; Kether (crown) being the highest and Malkut the lowest representing the earth realm. Shekinah resides in Malkut meaning Kingdom, the lowest of the ten Sephirot of the Tree of Life. Malkut represents the same principle as the first Chakra Muladhara (Earth Chakra) related to the consciousness of the material world. It appears, that the Shekinah from the Cabalistic perspective is the dwelling or vehicle of God, which he uses to ascend and descend the realms of the ten Sephirot represented by the Tree of Life. In its active role Shekinah is considered the Angel of liberation for human consciousness, placed just beneath the realm of God from the point of view of human salvation. Shekinah is a mediating consciousness between the infinitude of God and the limited human awareness.

The brain
The brain is the central organ of the nervous system and together with the spinal cord create the communication network of the body. This amazing organ (the brain) plays a role in every physical function of the body and controls our thoughts, memory, speech and movements. It consists of the forebrain (cerebrum), midbrain (brainstem) and hindbrain (cerebellum). Activities such as processing, integrating and coordinating information received from the sense organs and the functional and movement instructions sent to the rest of the body depend on the brain.

The brain is located in the head and protected by the bones of the skull and the spinal cord is located in the spine and protected by the vertebrae of the spinal column. The thalamus is the information gateway between the brain and the spinal cord. There are four cavities (ventricles) located within the brain, in a healthy person they are full of cerebral spinal fluid (CSF). Most of this fluid is produced by the choroid plexus, a plexus of cells that arises from the highly vascularised, loose connective tissue called the tela choroidea found in all of the ventricles. The CSF flows within and around the brain and spinal cord to help cushion them and protect them from injury. This circulating fluid is constantly being absorbed and replenished throughout one's life. There are billions of nerve cells (neurones) or grey matter and billions of nerve fibres (axons and dendrites) or white matter contained in the human brain.

Intelligence, creativity, emotion and memory are just a few things of the many the brain is constantly performing. The cerebrum is the largest part of the brain and is made up of the right and the left hemispheres, which are separated by a large bundle of myelinated nerve fibres called the corpus callosum. This bundle of nerve fibres allows communication between the right and left sides of the brain. The brain is also responsible for interpreting touch, vision, hearing, speech, reasoning, emotions, learning and movement. The cerebellum, known as the little brain is located in the back part of the head, under the cerebrum and is responsible for the coordination of muscle movement, posture and balance. The Brainstem is the relay centre connecting the cerebrum and cerebellum to the spinal cord. It is responsible for automatic functions such as breathing, heart rate, body temperature, wake and sleep cycles, digestion, sneezing, coughing, vomiting and swallowing.

The corpus callosum acts as the connector for exchanging information between the brain hemispheres. It ensures that both sides of the brain can communicate and transfer motor, sensory, and cognitive information between the brain hemispheres. Each hemisphere controls movement and feeling in the opposite side of the body. In general, the left hemisphere controls speech, comprehension, arithmetic and writing and the right hemisphere controls creativity, spatial abilities, artistic and musical skills. The left hemisphere is dominant in right handed people which make the majority of the population in the world. The theory is that if you are analytical and methodical in thinking you are left-brained, and if you tend to be more creative and artistic, you are right-brained.

According to an article published by Brain Plasticity / published online 2019 Dec 26; the practice of Yoga is linked to positive anatomical changes in the prefrontal cortex, hippocampus, amygdala, cingulate cortex, responsible for memory function as well as mood regulation. Another observation about Yoga is that whatever the yoga practitioner thinks, perceives and feels, whether intentionally or unconscious while practicing Yoga rewires the body-brain-mind system. Many yoga partitioners claim that practicing Yoga regularly has helped them improve their memory, coordination and reaction time.

From the Yoga perspective, the Crown Chakra (Sahasrara) at the top of the head rules the brain, nervous system and pituitary gland - the body's centres of knowledge and information. It is said that this Chakra is linked to our spiritual awareness, connection to the universe, and inner wisdom. When this Chakra is activated, it lifts and inspires the individual connecting him or her to the divine, the source of God. A sense of divinity and awareness that you are a soul within the human body becomes clear. This awareness strengthens the connection to the personal spirit or soul creating a sense of unity, power, and self knowledge.

From the Cabalistic perspective, Keter also known as Kether, meaning "Crown" is the topmost of the Sephirot of the Tree of Life. It is between Chokhmah and Binah and sits above Tiferet, which leads me to believe that Keter represents the "Corpus Calusum", which is a bundle of more than 200 million myelinated nerve fibres connecting the right and left brain hemispheres. In the stages of creation

Chokhmah (wisdom) is the upper most masculine element in the Godhead. It represents the origin of mental energy, thought and intellect originating from the right brain hemisphere. Binah (understanding), represents the analytical aspects of thought, represented by the left brain hemisphere, and the first female presence in the Tree of Life. And Tiferet (splendour) represents the spinal column and the force that integrates the masculine Chesed (compassion) represented by the right peripheral nervous system, and feminine Gevurah (strength) represented by the left peripheral nervous system. These two opposite forces, masculine and feminine are, respectively expansive (giving) and restrictive (receiving). When, combine and harmonised, they manifest the flow of Divine energy, and creation flowers forth.

The mind
The brain and the mind are not the same... the brain is the physical organ closely associated with the mind and consciousness. The mind is housed at least in part in the brain but it is independent from the body. It is invisible and it is the transcendent world of thought, feeling, attitude, belief and imagination. The stream of consciousness, sense impressions and mental phenomena the mind is continually creating, are always changing. These changes take place in the form of imagination, perception, thinking, feeling, intelligence, judgement, language and memory. When properly trained and develop this mental phenomena (the mind) can develop great faculties. The mind is that which enables us to have subjective awareness and intentionality towards our environment. It also allows us to perceive and respond to stimulation accordingly.

Regular yoga practice relaxes the mind, improves mental clarity, relieves stress, improves attention and sharpens concentration.

Other Mind Speculations:
Buddha, Zoroaster, Plato and Aristotle speculated that the mind was identical to the soul or spirit and had a direct link to life after death.
Descartes, placed the mind generally in the brain but, specifically in the pineal gland. Dualism claims that the mind exists independently of the brain.
Materialism claims that mental phenomena are identical to neuronal phenomena.

Idealism claims that only mental phenomena exist.
Medicine men, shamans, sadhus and even yogis have depended on herbs and other drugs to change the function of their brain and reach greater depths into their minds during their spiritual or shamanic rituals.

Studies have revealed that taking hallucinogenic drugs can significantly altered the electrical activity in the brain. Taking hallucinogenic drugs showed a substantial, drop in alpha waves, the brain's dominant electrical rhythm when we are awake and an increase of the short-lived theta brainwaves typically associated with deep relaxation, sleeping or dreaming. The theta waves are strong during internal focus, meditation, prayer, and spiritual awareness. They are very significant during the state between wakefulness and sleep, and closely connected to our subconscious mind.

Biomechanics in yoga

The human body, is made of four main elements: oxygen, carbon, hydrogen and nitrogen, with 60% in the form of water and the rest in the form of organic components such as: lipids, proteins, carbohydrates and nucleic acids. These elements form all the tissue types that constitute the human body, which include: epithelial, bone, muscle, nerve and connective tissue. The composition of these tissues form the different organ systems that account for the human body. Each system is responsible for a specific task to keep the body functioning smoothly. For example the respiratory system helps you breathe; the circulatory system helps your body tissues get enough oxygen and nutrients, and helps them get rid of waste products; the nervous system transmits signals to and from different parts of your body; and the musculoskeletal system is responsible for movement, support, protection, heat generation, and blood circulation within your body.

The musculoskeletal system is responsible for the body's biomechanics, which is the study of movement of the individual tissues and architecture of the human body. The structures that form the musculoskeletal system include: bones, ligaments, cartilage, tendons, connective tissue, nerves, muscles, and joints. During movement, in general the skeletal muscles pull on the bones causing the joints to move, which affect all the other tissues surrounding the joint. In the practice of Yoga, specially Yoga Asanas (postures), correct movement is essential for a good outcome and generate the desired benefits. The basic components of biomechanics are motion, force, momentum, levers, and balance which all are crucial components in the practice of Yoga postures. In Yoga, motion is referred to the movement through space of the body from the start to the completion of each individual posture. Speed defines to how fast you move into the posture, and acceleration defines how hard you push as you enter and hold the posture. And force meaning to push or pull during the practice of postures that causes the body to speed up, slow down, stop, or change direction which is crucial in the practice of Yoga.

The skeleton provides the framework for the muscles and the other soft tissues, including blood vessels, nerves, tendons, and tissues surrounding the bones and the joints. Together, they support the body's weight, maintain posture, and help the body move. In Yoga, biomechanics provides information that helps analyse the movements of the body during the practice of postures, which helps improve effectiveness and decrease the risk of injury. How the movement is analysed falls on a continuum between a qualitative analysis and a quantitative analysis. Qualitative methods allows the exploration of ideas and experiences during the practice of the postures in more detail. And quantitive methods allow to systematically measure variables such as modifications of the postures as a staring point for further investigation into what's the most appropriate practice method for the individual. The musculoskeletal system is responsible for posture and the internal and external movements of the body. In the practice of Yoga postures, some of the body movements can be very complicated which depend on the many interrelated muscles and other tissues responsible for their function. Moving the body and body parts in a precise manner during the practice of postures is essential for good biomechanics and precise body movements. Some of the basic principles in biomechanics, essential to know and apply in the practice of Yoga postures include: stability, effort, velocity, linear motion, angular motion and momentum. By understanding these principles and knowing how the body naturally wants to move the student can remove stress and pressure from the bones, joints, muscles and ligaments during the practice of postures, including during the practice of challenging ones.

The body depends on the muscular system to generate the active force required to execute the precise body movements. And for any physical movement to be generated the brain and the nervous system must command the skeletal muscles to act. The control of the skeletal muscles also known as "voluntary muscles" depend on a mind-body connection based on neural pathways made up of neurotransmitters, hormones and other chemicals. These chemical messengers are molecules used by the nervous system to transmit messages between neurones or from neurones to muscles.

Brain-mind and muscle connection
The biggest part of the brain is the cerebrum, is the thinking part and controller of the body's skeletal muscles. These muscles can be consciously control and commanded at will, any time the person feels like moving a body part. A neglected body can cause misalignment and weakness of these muscles compromising personal biomechanics which in turn will increase the wear and tear at the spine, making it fragile and prone to injury. The skeletal muscles are part of the musculoskeletal system which forms the framework of the human body. The tendons, ligaments and fibrous tissue bind the different body parts together creating stability. Good biomechanics can keep the musculoskeletal system strong, flexible, active, allowing the individual to enjoy the things he or she likes doing in life longer.

Yoga practice can strengthen the mind-muscle connection, especially when mental focus is directed to the active muscular region when practicing Yoga postures. The practice of postures in combination with good mental focus help multiply stronger muscle fibres, especially when good dietary habits are been practiced. By consciously or unconsciously, contracting the muscles attached to the bones (skeletal muscles), will translate into body movements. Nearly all movement in the body is the result of muscle contractions, including the movement taking place in the internal organs and blood vessels. A greater and stronger number of muscle fibres participating during the muscular contraction will result in a better physical performance overall.

In physiology, muscle contraction does not necessarily mean the shortening of the muscle but the tension generated when the muscle is engaged. Muscle contraction is followed by muscle relaxation, which is when the muscle returns to their low tension-generating state. Muscle contraction begins when the nervous system generates a signal or impulse, known as action potential. This impulse travels through the nerve cells called motor neurones, the basic unites of the nervous system. The motor neurones of the spinal cord connected to muscles, glands and organs throughout the body, transmit impulses from the spinal cord to the skeletal and smooth muscle, such as the ones in the stomach. The motor neurones directly control all movements generated by the muscles.

Types of muscle contraction
In biology muscle contraction, means activating, sometimes referred to as "firing" the skeletal muscles. According to this thinking, muscle contraction does not necessarily mean that the entire muscle shortens. Consider the fact that muscles consist of thousands of cells controlled by the nervous system. When the nervous system signal is sent to a muscle, is only a portion of the cells that receive the signal. This causes the proteins (actin and myosin) inside the cell to become attracted to one another, creating a contraction. But, that does not necessarily mean, that the entirety of the muscle is contracting or shortening, instead it creates an increased tension in the muscle. In other words, shortening, lengthening, or keeping the same length during the movement, are all considered muscle contractions.

The following are examples of different types of muscle contraction:

1. Isometric muscle contraction; this is a muscular contraction in which the length of the muscle does not change. This type of contraction places tension on muscles without causing movement in the surrounding joints. Some examples of isometric exercises include the plank and glute bridges.

2. Isotonic muscle contraction; this type of contraction shorten the muscle at a constant tension. A good example is when the arms are raised above the head to reach up at the beginning of the Half Moon

series. To be able to move the humerus at the shoulder joint, the deltoid muscles have to contract and shorten.

3. Eccentric muscle contraction; during this type of contraction the muscles lengthen and stretch. Functionally the muscles performing this type of contraction create a resistance, like in the Hands to Feet pose where the hamstrings resist the pull of gravity as the upper body is bending forward. Another example is, lowering into the bottom of a pushup, where the pecs lengthen and control the speed of the descent, creates an eccentric contraction.

4. Concentric muscle contraction; this contraction is a type of muscle activation that causes tension on the muscle as it shortens. For example, the upward phase of a biceps curl is a concentric contraction.

Joints and skeletal movement

The adult human skeletal system has a complex architecture that include 206 named bones connected by cartilage, tendons and ligaments which end up forming three types of joints: immovable, slightly movable and freely movable. The skeleton provides the framework for the 600 muscles give or take and other soft tissue that support the body, maintain posture and movement. For movement to take place the activated muscles contract and pull on the joints, allowing the body to move. Injuries, disease and ageing can cause pain, stiffness and other problems that will eventually reduce physical mobility. The best way to maintain the skeletal system, including the soft tissues and specially the joints responsible for movement in good working condition is to live an active and healthy life style.

The joints are classified by the material holding the ends of the bones together, their range of motion and function. This classification define the degree or lack of movement each individual joint allows for. Ageing and injuries play an important role in the health and mobility of the joints. As the synovial fluid (lubricating fluid) inside the skeletal joints decreases or dries up the joints become stiffer and less movable and the cartilage becomes thinner. Ageing does a number on the ligaments, tendons and muscles as well, they get shorter and stiffer which leads to the loss of flexibility, making the joint feel stiff and painful.

Studies have shown that the practice of Yoga can reduce joint pain by improving joint flexibility and function. The simple movements in the Yoga postures increase lubrication around the joints by stimulating the synovial glands. Increased lubrication can help slow down the wear and tear of cartilage which is often the cause of arthritic pain. Practicing Yoga regularly improves muscle strength and joint flexibility, while boosting mood and controlling stress.

Joint classification

1. Fibrous or immovable joints. These joints are defined as two or more bones closely connected that have no movement. The bones in the skull are one example.

2. Cartilaginous or slightly movable joints. The bones in these joints are held tightly together by cartilage that only limited movement is allowed. The spinal vertebrae are a good example.

3. Synovial or freely movable joints. These joints are the most movable and most common in the human body. The structural characteristic of these joints is the presence of a fluid-filled cavity where connecting surfaces of bones contact each other. This fluid is secreted into the joint space by the synovial glands originating from the synovial tissue. It allows the connecting bone surfaces which are covered with smooth articular cartilage to glide over each other with very little friction, making it easier to move. Articular cartilage can be damaged by injury or normal wear and tear, especially if the joint is out of alignment, making it difficult for good biomechanics. Symptoms of cartilage damage include: joint pain, swelling, stiffness, clicking or grinding sensation, joint locking, catching or giving way.

Each movement taking place at the synovial joints results from the contraction or relaxation of the muscles attached to the bones on either side of the joint. The degree and type of movement produced in the synovial joints is determined by their structure and type of joint in use. From all the different types of synovial joints, the ball-and-socket joint found in the hip and in the shoulders have the greatest range of movement. In other parts of the body, several joints may work together to produce a particular movement. Overall, each type of synovial joint is necessary to provide the body with great flexibility and mobility. If the synovial joints are not properly used and protected, they can be exposed to damage and the loss of flexibility, mobility and stability.

Staying mobile and keeping hydrated will keep the synovial fluid in the joints healthy. The right amount of synovial fluid will keep the ends of the bones, which are covered with cartilage sliding easily during body movement. Regular practice of Yoga can reduce joint pain, improve joint health, flexibility and function. The Yoga postures can increase lubrication in the joints and slowdown the breakdown of cartilage, especially when biomechanics and proper body movements are applied during their practice.

Muscular control

All physical movement is planned, controlled, directed and executed by the motor cortex. This is the region of the cerebral cortex involved in the execution of all voluntary body movements. The motor cortex on the right side of the brain is responsible for sending electrical signals through the spinal cord and peripheral nerves to the muscles on the left side of the body, making them contract. And the motor cortex on the left side of the brain is responsible for sending signals and firing up the muscles on the right side of the body. The sensory and motor information sent by the brain to the muscles move through descending cortical pathways. And ascending information sent by the muscles to the brain move through the peripheral pathways that tell the brain but especially the cerebellum where and how the arm, leg or any other part of the body should move. While the brain's motor system is contained mostly in the frontal lobes, the cerebellum located at the back of the brain beneath the occipital lobe is responsible for "fine tuning" movement and balance. The cerebellum is also called the "little brain" due to its many similarities with the cerebrum, the main part of the brain. The "little brain" is responsible for making postural adjustments in order to maintain balance and coordinate movement. Complicated movements require a greater number of muscles to work in coordination to execute the movement. To maintain a healthy brain is important to exercise regularly, get plenty of sleep, eat a healthy diet, stay mentally active and remain socially active.

The application of biomechanics and proper body movements during the practice of Yoga postures is essential to achieve good results. Once the ideal movement has been achieved, then it needs to be practiced frequently to maintain good form and get powerful results. Improper form may be targeting unintended muscle groups causing the joints and other soft tissues in the body to unwanted results and premature damage. The better the form the better the results in Yoga. Using good techniques is beneficial because it promotes higher performance and reduces the risk of injury. Yoga practitioners need to develop the skills necessary to perform the correct movements individual Yoga postures require for best results.

CENTRAL AXIS & MOVEMENT PLANES

The central axis of the human body is an imaginary line passing through the vertical centre from the head to the feet. It is the centreline from which the body initiates movement to the sides (lateral flexion), back (extension), forward (flexion) and rotation to the right or left side. Development of the body in most animals, including the human body takes place in a nearly symmetrical fashion around the central axis of the body. (The second cervical vertebra of the spine is also called axis. It is attached to the atlas or first cervical vertebra which carries and pivots the head.) This imaginary line (central axis) is created by the intersection of three imaginary planes (movement planes), which divide the body into front and back halves (coronal plane), left and right halves (sagittal plane), and top and bottom halves (transverse plane). The central axis is the imaginary centre line and reference point for the proportional distribution of weight exerted on the ground by the body while standing, walking, sitting, doing Yoga, or any other physical activity.

Coronal plane

The coronal plane is also called the frontal plane, divides the body into front and back sections. It is named after the coronal sutures of the human skull. The only movements possible in this plane are "abduction" and "adduction". Abduction is the movement of the torso or any other body part away from the axis. Adduction is the movement of the torso or body part toward the axis. The group of muscles engaged in abduction are assisted by the antagonistic muscles responsible for adduction and vice versa. For example; when you take a step to your right side, the movement of the leg is considered "abduction" and when you bring the step back toward the axis is considered "adduction". Or when you bend the torso to the right or the left side, away from the axis is considered "abduction" and when you return the torso back towards the axis is considered "adduction".

Sagittal plane

The sagittal plane is also know as the longitudinal plane, extending front and back. It divides the body into right and left halves. The name of this plane comes from the sagittal suture of the skull. The movements taking place within the trajectory of this plane are extension and flexion. Extension is the movement of the torso away from the central axis towards the back, back bends are a good example of this movement. Straightening the legs, arms, fingers and even toes is also called extension.

Flexion is the forward movement of the torso, forward bends are good examples of this movement. Bending the knees, elbows, fingers and toes is also called flexion. The angle between two body parts is reduced during flexion and the angle between two body parts is increased during extension. These two movements work hand in hand as well; when the torso is in extension, the back muscles are compressed supporting most of the body's weight and the front muscles are stretched out in opposition to assist and support the movement. And when in flexion the front muscles are compressed as the back muscles stretched to assist and support the movement as well. All the movements that require bending back or bending forward are done along the trajectory of sagittal plane.

Transverse plane

The transverse plane is also called the axial or X-Z plane. It is a flat, horizontal plane which divides the body into upper and lower halves. Twisting or rotational movements take place within this plane. The transverse plane is perpendicular to the coronal and sagittal planes and the point in the body where the three planes intersect, is consider the body's centre of gravity. When standing up in the Anatomical Position, the body's centre of gravity is found slightly forward of the first or second sacral segment (sacrum) of the spinal column. The sacrum is near the base of the spine, according to Yoga philosophy it is the protective place where the Goddess Kundalini is found, coiled up in her sleep.

Together with the ilium, ischium and pubis the sacrum form the pelvic crown which protects the reproductive organs and organs of waste elimination. During twisting of the torso the internal organs in the pelvic, abdominal, thoracic and throat are stimulated. Twists penetrate deep into the body's core which helps the detoxification of the body and increase its metabolic functions. Using the planes as the standard for complex physical movements will ensure proper physical symmetry and stronger concentration. It is important to follow the trajectory of the planes and respect personal physical limitations to stay properly aligned during the practice of Yoga postures. This is done to prevent over or under stretching, forcing or improperly twisting during the practice of Yoga postures.

MOVEMENT PLANES & TYPES YOGA POSITIONS:

"J" - Shaped Spine

Even though the J-shaped spine has been featured in most Greek sculptures, Esther Gokhale introduced it to the modern world in her method. She stresses that a posture with J-shaped spine is the ideal form, created to reposition the pelvis, knees, back, shoulders, and neck to improve the overall body's performance. By elongating the spine and lessening the burden on the lower back, while sitting, standing, laying down, bending over, and walking will prevent repetitive strain injuries. These type of injuries can happen during the practice of Yoga, work or in any other physical activity due to poor posture.

For the human, upright standing position the "J" shaped spine position is fundamental for a healthy, well aligned body. In this position, the skeleton is properly aligned with the body's central axis and the earth's centre of gravity which leads to less effort and energy consumption. The "J" shaped spine position also supports the back and abdominal muscles creating more space in the thorax for the lungs and the heart. More space allows these organs to function better. Also adopting the "J" shaped spine position will prevent back problems, which can be painful and limiting. One of the many benefits of having excellent posture is the ability to enjoy an active lifestyle without injuries for a much longer lifespan.

Standing "J" Shaped spine technique:
1. Stand with feet slightly apart
2. Push pelvis slightly back and raise breast bone so the abdominal cavity opens up.
3. Tuck chin slightly in and align head and shoulders.
4. Keep shoulders relaxed and slightly back.
5. Make sure you are standing perfectly aligned within the "Movement planes".

The anatomical position

In humans, the anatomical position is standing upright, ideally with a "J" shaped spine, along their central axis and movement planes. Stand with feet slightly apart in the J-shaped spine position, relax the arms down at your sides, turn palms to face towards the front and keep breast bone lifted forward. Keep legs straight, head levelled and ears aligned with the shoulders. In biomechanics, this position is used to identify and describe the relation and function of the different body parts in reference to one another. The anatomical position can be very helpful in realigning the body with the earth's centre of gravity which helps take pressure away from the joints. When the body is inline with the force of gravity, instead of fighting it, it moves in sink with it, which results in less energy consumption, better performance and more control. The terms used in biomechanics to describe the four sides of the body in relation to the movement planes are: anterior (front), posterior (back), medial (middle), lateral (right or left sides).

In Hatha Yoga the anatomical position is the best position to prepare the body and mind for the movements required to do all standing Yoga postures. It is a basic position that should be done before and after each and every standing posture. The anatomical position is essential as preparation for the understanding and execution of the movement planes to generate correct and safe joint movement during the practice of all the standing yoga positions.

Since I, personally started standing with the "J" shaped spine during the anatomical position before and after each one of the standing postures my Yoga practice improved, greatly. Practicing the anatomical position regularly gave me a new way of looking at my Yoga practice. And after 45 years, plus and thousands and thousands of hours of intense practice, I can proudly say that my body feels better than ever. I believe, following these basic anatomical principles prevented me from experiencing common injuries experienced by many Yoga practitioners such as: knee, back, shoulder or spinal injuries due to poor posture and poor biomechanics.

Backbends (extension)

Extension or back bends follow the trajectory of the sagittal plane, which runs front to back. Externally, the targeted focus of extensions is the compression of the back muscles, assisted by the antagonistic front muscles. Internally, this movement reverses the natural tendencies of the spinal column to be in constant flexion. The regular practice of extensions help decompress the movable regions of the spinal column, relieving pressure and pain. These movable regions include the lumbar (lower spine), thoracic (upper spine) and cervical (neck). There are 23 discs located in between the movable spinal vertebrae. These discs provide three primary functions: they absorb spinal shocks, hold the vertebrae together, and allow mobility in the spine. The coccyx and sacrum, the lowest two parts of the spine are fused vertebrae and have no mobility. The lumbar and cervical regions have the greatest mobility and the thoracic region has limited mobility because of the ribs which form a cage to protect the organs in the chest. By pushing the vertebral discs forward during extension, strengthen the back muscles and help prevent spinal discs bulging or herniation.

The combination of spinal strength, flexibility and balance made it possible for the human body to be able to stand upright and walk. But in the same way the human spine unfolded to allow humans to do the things we do; unnatural, misaligned ways, time and wear and tear will shut down the spine once again. To prevent this from happening prematurely, Hatha Yoga have include many extension poses in its systems. Extension poses are one of the best antidotes to prevent premature ageing over all.

Forward bends (flexion)

Flexion or forward bending poses are done within the trajectory of the sagittal plane as well, the same as the extension postures. The targeted focus of flexion postures is the stimulation of the internal organs, including organs in the pelvic, abdominal and thoracic regions. Standing flexion postures or standing forward bends are considered semi-inverted positions. They turn the upper body and internal organs including the lungs, heart and brain upside down. Changing the position of these organs, changes the pressure they receive which helps bring changes to the overall circulation in the body. This semi-inverted postures improve the blood pressure and circulation to areas in the body where circulation is normally hard to reach due to our upright position. The safest way to do standing forward bends is to move from the hip joints, with a straight, flat back. Keeping a flat back during flexion postures will keep the front edges of the vertebrae away from each other and the spinal discs forward, towards the front of the spine which is the ideal place for them to be.

The floor flexion or forward bends can be done with a flat or round back, for example; during the Separate Legs Heat to Knee the back is rounded and during the Stretching pose the back should be flat. The flexion poses done with a flat back require the movement to take place at the level of the hips and postures done with a round back, the movement is based on rounding the spine which brings the edges in the front part of the vertebrae closer together. Rounding the spine helps stimulate the central nervous system and all the internal organs. Both standing and floor forward bends improve flexibility in the back and leg muscles. Doing forward bends correctly will strengthen pelvic, spinal, back and abdominal muscles.

Side bends (lateral flexion)

Lateral flexion or side bending postures are done within the trajectory of the coronal plane, extending to the right or left sides of the body. The primary focus in this movement is to improve the flexibility in the spine and the ribcage. Lateral flexion also changes the position and pressure of the internal organs, especially in the chest cavity. For example, during flexion to the right side, the torso bends, creating a right side compression, changing the pressure and circulation of the lungs, heart and other soft tissues in the thoracic region. The antagonistic muscles on the opposite side stretch and assist the right lateral movement and vice versa when the movement is done over towards the left side. Practicing side bends will also help strengthen the lateral muscles, tendons and ligaments in the spine, rib cage and hips. It is important to strive for proper alignment to generate a solid side compression when doing lateral flexion.

Twisting poses

Twisting postures follow the trajectory of the transverse plane during this movement. B.K.S. Iyengar described twisting postures as; "Squeeze and Soak" action. He also said, "The organs are compressed during twists, pushing out blood filled with metabolic byproducts and toxins. When released the fresh blood flows in, carrying oxygen and the building blocks for tissue healing. Twists stimulate circulation and have a cleansing and refreshing effect on the internal organs and associated glands".

Inversion poses

Inversion poses move the legs within the sagittal plane, bringing the body to an up side down position, along the central axis of the body. During inversions the heart is placed at a higher level than the head therefore increasing blood pressure and circulation to the upper part of the body, especially to the brain. Placing the body up-side down helps circulate blood back to regions where circulation is hard to reach due to our up-right position and the effects the force of gravity has on the body. Up-side down body postures stimulate the lymphatic system which helps flush out toxins, excess proteins and bacteria out of the body. Mentally, this type of postures help build a strong sense of self confidence.

Meditative postures

In the meditative postures the spine should be centred within the central axis of the body to reinforce the body-mind connection. The ideal postures for meditation are usually sitting but sometimes standing or reclining positions. The best known postures for meditation are the postures in the lotus series, that include Pranasana (life pose), Sukhasana (easy pose), Siddhasana (success in meditation pose), Ardha-padmasana (half lotus pose) and Padmasana (lotus pose). It is essential to keep the back in an upright position, perpendicular to the floor during the practice of these postures. By keeping the spine straight, the energy connects with and enhances the energy of the chakra system. Other meditation postures include kneeling positions or sitting on a chair with the spine erect. The aim in meditation is to focus on the breath first, followed by a body scanning to help lessen anxiety-based tension that may be held in body without even knowing that it is there. And finally the mind should be focus on one single part in the body, this point can be any of the body plexuses called chakras along the spinal column or the third eye in the middle of the forehead. Meditation prepares the person to respond, rather than react in difficult situations.

Relaxation postures

The main relaxation posture in yoga is called "Savasana" (corpse pose) which is done within the trajectory of the sagittal plane. This relaxation posture helps to consciously release the muscular grip caused by stress and muscular tension. It also helps loose and dismantle mental and emotional tension and strain. Relaxation postures overall help overcome physical discomfort caused by anxiety and fear. Deep relaxation affects different aspects of the person including the ability to be calm, focused, balanced and feel good about oneself. Relaxation postures are essential to get the full therapeutic benefits from the practice of Yoga overall.

THE RESPIRATORY SYSTEM & PRANAYAMA

Breath awareness (pranayama) is the key component during the practice of yoga postures. This awareness and control will make an efficient use of the abdominal and diaphragmatic muscles and improve the respiratory system. The respiratory system is a biological system consisting of airways, lungs and muscles in the human body, together they generate the functions needed to keep the organism alive. Young people, for the most part are endowed with reasonably healthy organisms that function well but as they grow older the organs slowly begin to shutdown until the end of life.

By increasing oxygen intake, improving lung elasticity, capacity and efficiency the respiratory system will stay healthy late into one's life. Pranayama, this ancient breath technique is based on a series of breathing exercises involved in controlling the breath in different styles and lengths. The practice of these techniques bring clarity of the mind, increases lung capacity, strengthen will power, reduce stress and anxiety and improve inner and outer health.

The main objective of pranayama is to increase the oxygen intake of the body. The delivery of oxygen rich blood to the cells in the brain, heart, lungs and digestive organs enabling them to work better and longer therefore improving the practitioners overall health. All the cells in the body absorb oxygen to stay healthy, reproduce and function efficiently before dying. As they perform their work, the cells produce carbon dioxide (CO_2), an odourless, colourless, waste product in the body. The blood carries this waste gas to the lungs to be breathed out and breathe in oxygen for as long as we are alive. When the mechanism to maintain this balance no longer functions efficiently, severe symptoms such as difficulty in breathing, respiratory failure, seizures and even coma can happen. Healthy breathing not only keeps us alive and functioning smoothly, it is one of the greatest pleasures in life.

During inhalations the respiratory system takes air into your lungs, then the oxygen in the air is taken by the alveoli to the alveolar walls through the capillaries (tiny blood vessels) lining to be absorbed by the bloodstream. Once in the bloodstream, the oxygen gets picked up by the haemoglobin (Hb) in the red blood cells, the iron-containing oxygen-transport in the body. At the level of each individual cell, the oxygen is exchanged for the waste gas CO_2. The blood stream then carries this waste gas back to the lungs where it is removed from the bloodstream and then exhaled out of the body. This function is automatically performed, it is a vital process, called gas exchange. During the exhalation, the diaphragm moves upward and the chest wall muscle relax, causing the chest cavity to get smaller, pushing the air carrying carbon dioxide out of the respiratory system through the nose and mouth. Correct breathing involves abdominal, thoracic and clavicular inhalations and exhalations.

The primary objective in the pranayama method is to gain conscious control over the breathing process, especially during the practice of Yoga poses and meditation. The nose, mouth, pharynx, larynx, trachea, bronchi and bronchioles are the airways which carry the air between the lungs and the exterior of the body. The health and well being of any breathing organism is highly dependent on the following functions related to breathing:
    1. Gas exchange - oxygen for carbon dioxide.
    2. Breathing - moving air in and out of the body.
    3. Sound production - voice.

4. Olfactory assistance - sense of smell.

5. Protection - from dust and microbes entering the body with the help of mucus, cilia and coughing.

6. Metabolism - biochemical process of combining nutrients with oxygen.

All living, breathing organisms depend on the chemical reactions taking place by the gas exchange of oxygen for carbon dioxide within all the living organisms. This exchange of gases will continue for as long as the organism is alive. For this exchange to take place smoothly, the respiratory system works twenty-four - seven, even during sleep. The respiratory system, together with the circulatory system provide the oxygen to the cells during inhalation. The waste products produced by the cells during the body's metabolism is removed from the blood stream during the exhalation. The health of the organism depends on this gas exchange.

All the chemical reactions in the body, including those that use oxygen and create carbon dioxide are considered part of the body's metabolism. Therefore, oxygen and carbon dioxide play an important role in both respiration and metabolism. The metabolic reactions at the cellular level are also known as cellular respiration, a processes that uses glucose to produce adenosine triphosphate (ATP), an organic compound the body uses for energy. This processes to convert nutrients into chemical energy, releases metabolic waste which is excreted from the body in form of water-solutes through the excretory organs including tubules and kidneys, with the exception of CO2. The elimination of these waste products enables the chemical homeostasis of the body, responsible for the steady internal, physical and chemical balance of the living-organism.

ANATOMY OF MOVEMENT

The brain is the command centre of the body, together with the spinal cord form the central nervous system (CNS). The spinal cord is a column of nerve tissue that runs from the base of the skull down through the centre of the spinal column to the lower back. It is a delicate structure that contains nerve bundles and neurones (nerve cells) that carry messages from the brain to the peripheral nervous system (PNS). The peripheral nervous system is composed of all the nerves that branch out from the central nervous system and extend to the different parts of the body, including sense organs, muscles and glands. It is the connection between the central nervous system (brain and the spinal cord), to the rest of the body. The peripheral nervous system plays a key role in both sending information from the different areas of the body back to the brain, as well as carrying out commands from the brain to the different parts of the body.

It has being estimated that the human body has an average of 86 billion neurones (brain cells) and 85 billion non-neuronal cells. Neurones are the fundamental units of the brain and the nervous system. They are responsible for receiving sensory information from the external world, for sending motor commands to the muscles, and transforming and relaying the electrical signals at every step of the way in between. The neurones interact closely with the non neuronal cells classified as glial cells. The glial cells provide support and protection to the neurones, maintain homeostasis, clean up debris, and form myelin, a protective layer that wraps around the axons of the neurones. Glial cells basically work to care for the neurones and the environment they live in.

Both the brain and the spinal cord are protected by bone: the brain by the bones of the skull, and the spinal cord by the vertebrae, a set of ring-shaped bones. They are both cushioned by layers of membranes called meninges, and cerebrospinal fluid. The brain is divided into three parts: fore brain, midbrain and hindbrain. It is an electrical power house, made of soft tissue containing neurones (nerve cells) and non-neuronal cells. And the spinal cord is a cylindrical structure that runs through the centre of the spine, from the brainstem to the low back. It is a delicate structure comprised of three different parts: cervical (neck), thoracic (chest), and lumbar (lower back) regions. The spinal cord contains bundles of neurones (nerve cells) that carry messages from the brain to the rest of the body. This amazing cord is connected to the brain through the brainstem consisting of three structures as well: the medulla oblongata, the pons, and the midbrain.

The neurones in the frontal lobes part of the forebrain are responsible for many different functions including motor skills, such as voluntary movement, speech, intellectual and behaviour functions. The neurones in the motor cortex, part of the frontal lobes generate the signals that trigger movement in different parts of the body. Movement is a fundamental aspect of life, it affects everything, from circulation to digestion, to metabolism, and even the immunity of the body. With movement the body regulates hormone activity, detoxification and respiration as well.

The neurones in the medulla oblongata, the lowest part of the brainstem play an essential role in transmitting signals between the spinal cord and the higher parts of the brain. These neurones are responsible for regulating breathing, heart rhythm, blood pressure and swallowing. The medulla oblongata is connected to the spinal cord through the foramen magnum an opening at the bottom of the skull. Just above the medulla is the pons, a broad horseshoe-shaped mass responsible for relaying impulses from the motor cortex to the cerebellum, medulla, and thalamus. The cerebellum is located at the back of the head, just above and behind where the spinal cord connects to the brain.

The neurones in the cerebellum are responsible for muscle control and movement that include walking, posture, balance, coordination, eye movements, and speech. The thalamus is a small structure within the brain located just above the brainstem between the cerebral cortex and the mid brain. It is considered the body's information relay station. Its neurones process and relay the information from the senses (except smell) to the cerebral cortex for interpretation. The neurones in the cerebral cortex (the outer layer of the brain that lies on top of the cerebrum) are responsible for higher-level processes of the brain, including language, memory, reasoning, learning, decision- making, emotion, intelligence and personality.

At the beginning of any physical movement, the motor neurones of the brain first send a signal to the motor neurones of the spinal cord, the motor neurones of the spinal cord send the signal to the motor neurones of the peripheral nervous system to tell the body part to move. Then the neurones from the peripheral nervous system sends back the status report to the brain by relaying information via the sensory nerves. Each neurone has a long cord that snakes away from the cell known as the axon, which transmits the electrochemical signals through which neurones communicate. Axons of the peripheral nervous system run together in bundles called fibres, and multiple fibres form the nerve, the cable of the electric circuit. The nerves, which contain connective tissue and blood vessels, reach out to the muscles, glands and organs in the entire body.

The peripheral nervous system is a network of nerves that branch off from the left and right sides of the spinal cord through openings between each vertebra on the spinal canal. These nerves spread in pairs throughout the entire body to deliver commands from the brain and spinal cord to and from different parts of the body. They are classified as afferent nerves, from the Latin "afferre" "to bring towards" and efferent nerves, that means "to bring away from". The neurones from the afferent nerves bring information to the central nervous system (brain & spinal cord). And the neurones from the efferent nerves transmit the signals originating in the central nervous system to the organs and skeletal muscles to execute voluntary movements, such as lifting the arms above the head and interlacing the fingers.

All of the body's voluntary movements are controlled by the brain. One of the brain areas most involved in controlling these movements is the motor cortex. The motor cortex is located in the rear portion of the frontal lobe, just before the central sulcus (furrow) that separates the frontal lobe from the parietal lobe. There is a theory, that in all voluntary movements the initial action takes place in the supplementary motor areas (SMA) in both cerebral hemispheres. It has been shown that the SMA, particularly its connectivities to the basal ganglia (a group of subcortical nuclei responsible for motor control) and the cerebellum are active in the programming of a voluntary movements.

Thus by its neuronal connectivities the SMA is able to bring about the desired movement. The mental act of intention plays an important role in generate neural actions in the SMA that eventually lead to the intended movement.

Specialised, voluntary movements play important roles in physical activities designed to enhance or maintain physical and mental fitness, overall health and wellness. These activities, including sports, dance and yoga which are performed for different reasons such as: to help growth, develop muscles, improve strength, maintain flexibility, enhance physical and mental balance, boost the cardiovascular system and enrich the capacity of the brain to mention a few. Physical activity supply nerve cells (neurones) with oxygen, promote the production of new cells, and aid in creating strong synapses. It is the place of transmission of electric nerve cells (neurones) between another cell, gland or muscles cell. Movement in general enhances the health of the brain as well as the health of the body by improving overall circulation. Having better circulation means better delivery of oxygen and nutrients to the 86 billion neurones (nerve cells) and the 85 billion glial cells that constitute the human brain. Physical activity not only improve brain structure, cognitive performance, attention and memory, but the all around health of the human being.

THE SKELETON & SKELETAL MUSCLES

206 bones, give or take form the human skeleton. It is the framework that supports the human body in the upright position and forms the armour that protects the heart, lungs and brain. The shape and placement of the human skull, rib cage, pelvis and scapula bones as well as the bones of the extremities play a direct role on one's ability to move. The two distinct skeletal unites that constitute the human skeleton are the axial skeleton and the appendicular skeleton. The axial skeleton is made up of the bones in the central axis of the body such as the skull, vertebral column, rib cage and sternum. The appendicular skeleton is made up of the bones of the arms, and legs, including hands and feet. The arms are attached to the sternum at the sternoclavicular joints and the legs to the sacrum at the sacroiliac joints. The sternoclavicular and sacroiliac joints are the areas where movement such as flexing, extending and rotating of the spine and extremities take place.

The skeletal muscles are attached by tendons to the bones of the skeleton. The cells of these muscles are much longer than in any other type of muscle tissue, and are defined as muscle fibres. Each skeletal muscle consists of thousands of

118

muscle fibres wrapped together by connective tissue. The individual bundles of muscle fibres in a skeletal muscle are called fascicle. These muscle fibres stretch out across the skeleton and when they contract cause the tendons to pull the attached bones generating movement. Tendons essentially work as levers to move the bones as the muscles contract or expand. Tendons are strong bands of dense, regular connective tissue stiffer than muscles and have tremendous amounts of strength. Skeletal muscles are found in the arms and legs, abdomen, back, neck and head. The reason these muscles are called skeletal muscles is because they are attached to the bones.

Skeletal muscles are also responsible for subtle movements that result from facial expressions such as eye movements, and respiration. In addition to movement, skeletal muscles also fulfil other important functions in the body, such as posture, joint stability, and heat production. Overall the skeletal system supports and gives structure to the body, and the muscular system allows for voluntary and involuntary physical movements. And the nervous system controls all the movements taken place in the body, including all the organ functions.

SEVEN PRINCIPLES OF MOVEMENT

Fetal movement can be felt as early as 16 weeks of pregnancy, from a flutter, kick, swish or roll. Generally an active baby is a healthy baby. The movement the baby generates in the womb helps promote healthy bone and joint development. Many babies learn to crawl between 7 months and ten months, crawling is considered the first form of independent movement. It helps the baby develop and enhance the vestibular/balance system, sensory system, cognition, problem solving skills, and coordination. As the child grows older he or she uses and moves his or her body in different ways to activate their brain. And the brain responds in full force allowing them to move in a variety of ways including crossing the midlines. Learning to cross all three lines, reaching top to bottom (transverse plane), left to right (coronal plane), and front to back (sagittal plane) demand coordination from both sides of he brain.

Regular physical movement is one of the most important things teenagers and adults can do for their health. By moving, the joints get more flexible and the muscles get stronger, which provide stability, balance and coordination. Movement also releases endorphins and help relieve stress and allows emotions to move through the body a lot easier. The endorphins released during movement will help the person feel healthier and think better. It is recommended to move for approximately three minutes at least every hour during the day to feel one's best. The structure of the human body allows for at least eight different basic movements that require the use of multiple joints, these movements include: pull, push, squat, lunge, hinge, extension, rotation and gait. These movements are the basis of every exercise there is, including sports, dance and specially Hatha Yoga. All the Yoga postures incorporate one or several of these movements.

1. Pull, this motion consists of pulling a weight towards the body or the body towards a thing or body part towards the midline, like in returning to the midline after the Lateral Half Moon. This movement can be a vertical (standing) such as a pull up or horizontal (laying on the floor) such as pulling the legs into the chest during the Wind Relieving pose. The main muscles being worked in these set of movements are the mid and upper back, biceps, forearms, back and part of the shoulders.

2. Push, this motion is the opposite of the movements base on pulling. Pushing movements involve thrusting a weight away from the body or the body away from an object or floor like in the practice of push-ups. There are many Yoga postures that use this movement such as Crow, Crain and Finger Stand. The muscles targeted are the chest, triceps, and front part of the shoulders.

3. Squat, this movement is one of the most complex movement the human body is capable of doing. There are several Yoga postures based on this type of movement, including Awkward and Toe Stand. The squat targets the glutes, core muscles, quadriceps and to a lesser degree the hamstring.

4. Lunge, this movement targets the lower extremities which places the body in a less stable position, like in the Warrior pose where one foot is further forward than the other. Since the position of the body is at a disadvantage stance, this movement demands greater concentration, flexibility, stability and balance. The lunge hits the glutes, quadriceps, core muscles, and hamstrings.

5. Hinge, this movement is executed by kicking the butt back and leaning the torso forward while maintaining a neutral spine, like in the Standing Hands to Feet pose or when picking up something from the floor. These movements stretches the posterior chain, which comprises the hamstring, glutes, and lower back.

6. Extension, this movement is performed by bending the torso back, like in all the back bent poses. It happens when the back muscles contract and the front muscles, including internal organs and the joints

of the spine stretch. This movement develop and strengthen the back muscles and improves body posture.

7. Rotation, this is unique movement in comparison from the other six movements because of the plane that it works in. The other movements involve moving forward and backward or side to side, yet rotation involves twisting at the core. This movement is underrated despite being essential for success in sports. There are several Yoga postures based on rotation. Rotation is also seen while throwing a ball, kicking a ball, changing directions while running and many other actions. The core, specifically the oblique muscles are the main contributors to this type of movement.

8. Gait, is a combination of multiple movements involving balance and coordination of the muscles so that the body is propelled forward in a rhythm like motion such as walking, jogging and jumping.

The practice of the Yoga postures is ruled by force, motion or movement and speed when entering, holding, and existing the poses. The proper management of these three basic fundamentals (force, motion & speed) is essential for the proper execution of the postures, in general. Since range of motion or degree of joint and muscle flexibility and muscular strength dictate the depth each individual can reach in each of the postures, the primary goal is to improve these two component of fitness in a gradual, cumulative and safe way. While holding the postures motionless and in complete stillness which is the ultimate aim in yoga, concentration and will power are essential.

Good skeletal, joint and muscular alignment for their proper development during the practice of postures depends in the right understanding and application of the movement planes; coronal, sagittal and transverse. The implementation of these planes will lead to good biomechanics which will improve physical effectiveness and will reduce or even eliminate the overall risk of injury.

Good understanding of these basic principles will help develop a solid, safe and sustainable Yoga practice. The proper application of these basic exercise fundamentals in the practice of Yoga postures is essential to get in better shape, improve physical fitness, performance and mental concentration.

BASIC TRAINING PRINCIPLES:

Yoga teachers should keep in mind that we all are unique individuals with slightly different responses to the movements each individual posture requires. It means that "One way of describing the pose does not work for all". The postures must be explained based on the fitness level or physical condition of the practitioner and not with a general descriptions based on a dialogue.

Individual differences should dictate the approach the practitioner should take when practicing the poses. Some of these physical differences have to do with body size and shape, genetics, injuries, chronic conditions and even gender. For example, older practitioners generally need to approach the postures slower than younger individuals due to their loss of strength, flexibility and balance. Also an older person needs more recovery time in between the postures than younger practitioners.

Another example is when a muscular person attempts to do postures that require flexibility and due to their muscular frame they have a greater challenge than a person with normal musculature.

1. Overload

The overload principle states that a greater than normal effort, stress or load on the body is necessary during the practice of Yoga to be able to improve. This workload needs to be increased according to the needs of the practitioner, for it to be effective. In order for the muscles, including the heart to be able to improve their level of fitness the Yoga practitioners must be gradually pushed. In Yoga the overload principle takes place when the effort is gradually increased against the resistance experienced during the practice of the postures. The practitioner needs to press on or overload beyond the comfort zone or what he or she is accustomed to, to be able to improve. This can be done by several different ways, for example: hold the posture longer than usual; increase the effort and intensity; or increment the number of repetitions when doing the posture.

2. Progression

The level of effort and intensity (overload) during the practice of Yoga should be gradual and systematic, increased over a period of time for best results. This is the safest and most effective approach to generate physical and mental benefits and improve the practitioner's fitness level without risk of injury. Keep in mind, that when the overload principle is not applied, improvement is unlikely, but when the overload principle is increased to quickly, it may result in injury or tissue damage. For example, the weekend practitioner who does one yoga class vigorously only on the weekends violates the principle of progression and most likely will expose himself to injury and not see any fitness gains.

The overload principle also addresses the need to rest and recover. That it is why during the standing postures the "Anatomical Position" is done, and during the floor postures "Savasana", also known as the Corpse pose is highly recommended. Progression without rest may result in exhaustion and injury. Training hard all the time, has the risk of overtraining and a decrease in fitness but not training hard enough may not produce any results. Finding the right timing, ideal pace and level of effort or overload during practice is essential for the very best results of each individual.

4. Adaption

The principle of adaption relates to the ability to adjust by increasing or decreasing physical effort while doing the postures. It is a way to learn to coordinate muscle movement and develop Yoga skills more efficiently. Adaption describes why beginners are often sore after their first Yoga session, but after a few days and weeks of regular practice, they have little if any soreness. The repetitive practice of the same exercise, over time will become second-nature and easier to perform that is what adaption means. Changing or incorporating a new exercise routines or sequence of Yoga postures may cause body soreness once again, until the new muscle groups or body parts get use to the new routine.

5. Use / Disuse

Use/disuse implies that when it comes to fitness, regular practice improves or maintains one's level of fitness. No practice will do the opposite, which leads to an unfit physical and mental condition. Proper use (exercise) of the body increases the number of cells and growth of the muscles (hypertrophy). And the disuse or lack of exercise decreases the muscular mass, number of cells, and even organ function (atrophy). That is why the physical level of fitness improves with regular practice and decreases when the person stops exercising.

6. Specificity

The specificity principle describes how physical benefits gained are specific to the type of training the person performs. For example, jogging regularly will improve performance as well as aerobic conditioning. Doing yoga regularly, will improve strength, flexibility and balance. Another important difference is that each Yoga posture is designed to target specific body parts therefore, they can be used as therapy or as a fitness program. Repeating the same physical activity or sequence of postures, over time will develop the specific areas targeted, and to be able to make more gains the overload principle is essential.

Understanding and applying effort, body movements, range of motion, and relaxation in combination with the six training principles mentioned above, will give the practitioner the greatest advantages in the fitness field. Within Hatha Yoga there are postures for every practitioner, some are easy and others difficult.

The easy postures work on areas of the practitioner's body that have being properly developed. The difficult ones work on the under or overly developed areas of the body.

There is a consensus in Yoga that to be able to properly balance the body, the practitioner needs to focus close attention to the difficult postures. The difficult postures will strengthen or stretch the joints, muscles, and other tissues preventing the practitioner from properly executing them. The regular practice of the difficult postures, in time will improve muscular balance, having good muscle balance will improve coordination, which will naturally improve the practitioner's ability to face challenging tasks with ease. This means improved agility, quicker reaction time, and overall performance.

CORE 26+ FOR PHYSICAL & MENTAL FITNESS

During the practice of the poses in this system, the anatomical position and the imaginary lines of the movement planes (coronal, sagittal & transverse) are essential. These conceptual lines must be followed to improve physical alignment, weight distribution and to effectively isolate the specific body parts (specificity) targeted by the postures. Side to side postures (lateral flexion) follow the trajectory of the coronal plane, this conceptual line divides the body into exact front and back halves. Extension postures (back bends) and flexion postures (forward bends) follow the trajectory of the sagittal plane, this line divides the body into exact right and left halves. And twisting postures follow the trajectory of the transverse plane which divides the body into top and bottom halves.

Understanding the personal axis, anatomical position and trajectories of the movement planes when entering, holding and exiting the poses will help build a safe, generative, sustainable and fun Yoga practice. The laws of movement, movement planes and the six training principles are the foundation for the mastery of Yoga postures.

During the practice of this system (Core26+), you will find easy and difficult postures. The easy postures will be targeting the structures of your body in good physical condition and the difficult ones will be focusing on the areas that need the most work. Understanding how your body wants to naturally move, and applying the anatomical position before and after every standing posture is essential for good results. The movement planes and the six training principles will help restore lost flexibility, strength and balance in a gradual progressive way. In general, during the practice of these Yoga postures "Never sacrifice alignment for depth". Do stay the course, even during your greatest challenge and in a short amount of time you will see and feel tremendous progress.

Difficult postures are essential to stretch tight areas, or strengthen weak and unstable ones to create a harmonious physical and mental balance. Learn to appreciate and love the challenge, take your time, be careful and keep one pointed focus when practicing.

Core 26 + is a beginners system, composed of 26 postures plus a few variations, the Standing Deep Breathing at the beginning and Kapalabhati at the end. The Standing Deep Breathing is a warm-up breathing exercise that helps prepare the muscles for movements required for the execution of the postures. The postures in the system are laid out in a way that will help condition the body, improve mind-body connection, enhance and maintain ultimate physical fitness, and overall health in a gradual, progressive and safe way. And Kapalabhati at the end is to detoxify the body in preparation for the deep relaxation taking place in "Savasana" which concludes the session.

Internally, the postures in Core26+ stimulate the flow of energy and blood circulation through compression, extension and twisting to all the internal organs in the body, including the brain in the skull, spinal cord in the spine, lungs and heart in the chest, digestive organs in the abdominal cavity, and organs of reproduction and elimination in the pelvic region. The skull, spine and rib cage are classified as the axial skeleton and the limbs and girdles in the shoulders and hips as the appendicular skeleton. The bones of the appendicular skeleton (extremities) are attached to the axial skeleton, together they form the skeleton of the human body. Good understanding of the axial and appendicular skeletons is essential to maintain good alignment and for proper execution of bio- mechanics during the practice of the Yoga postures.

Core 26 +, the list
In this each breathing exercise and postures are assigned a number to better understand the system.

   A. Standing Deep Breathing / Pranayama
     1. Lateral Half Moon - Parsvardhacandrasana
       1. Back bend - Ardhacandrasana / variation of Lateral Half Moon
     2. Hands to Feet - Padahastasana
     3. Triangle -Trikonasana
     4. Standing Separate Leg Head to Knee - Dandayamana Vibhakta Pada Janushirasana
     5. Awkward (three Parts) - Utkatasana
     6. Eagle - Garudasana
     7. Standing Head to Knee - Dandayamana Janushirasana
     8. Standing Bow - Dandayamana Dhanurasana
     9. Balancing Stick - Tuladandasana

10. Splits in the Air - Dandayamana Purna Janushirasana
11. Separate Leg Stretching - Dandayamana Vibhakta Pada Paschimottanasana
12. Tree - Tadasana
13. Corpse Pose - Savasana
14. Wind Removing - Pavanamuktasana (three Parts)
15. Cobra - Bhujangasana
16. Locust - Salabhasana (three Parts)
17. Full Locust - Purna Salabhasana
18. Bow - Dhanurasana
19. Half Tortoise - Ardha Kurmasana
20. Camel - Ustrasana
21. Rabbit - Sasangasana
22. Head to Knee - Janushirasana
23. Stretching - Paschimotthanasana
    1. Separate Leg Stretching - Vibhaktapadapascimottanasana
24. Upward Stretching - Utthitapascimottanasana
25. Happy Cow Face - Gomukhasana
26. Spinal Twist - Ardha Matsyendrasana

B. Kapalbhati - Breathing Exercise

In the description of the postures, the breathing exercises are classified by letters, and the Half Moon series as one which includes three different postures.

A. Standing Deep Breathing

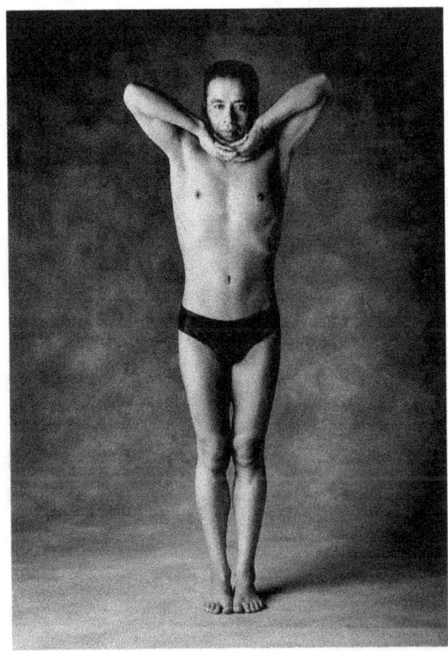 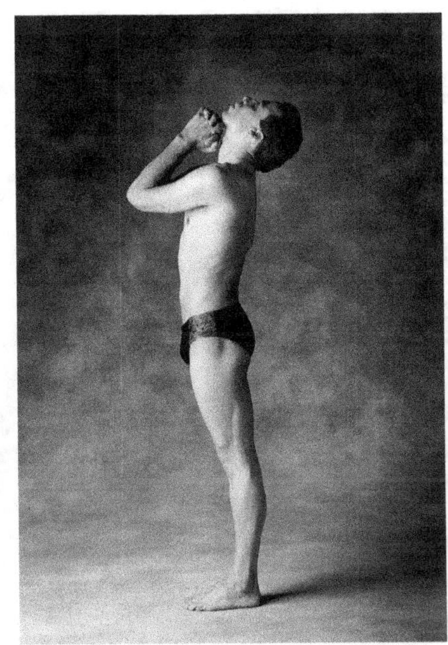

1. Stand tall in the Anatomical Position.

2. Interlace your fingers, place them under your chin, lift your head, bring elbows close together and inhale through your nose.

3. Exhale through your nose and simultaneously bring your head down as you raise your elbows up towards your ears and pause for one to two seconds.

4. Inhale through your nose as you raise and extend your head back and bring your elbows forward and close together and pause for one or two seconds.

5. Keeping back straight, exhale as you lower your head forward and raise your elbows up toward your ears, and pause.

6. Repeat inhalation and exhalation for ten times before lowering your arms down.

"Breathing is the greatest pleasure in life"- *Giovanni Papini*

1. Lateral Half Moon

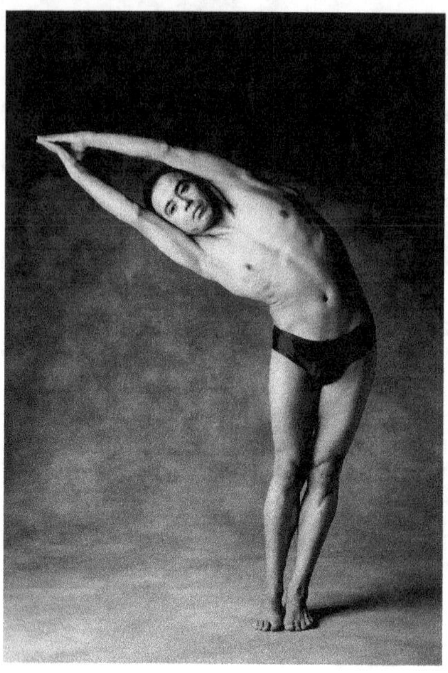

1. Stand tall in the Anatomical Position breathing naturally.

2. Within the coronal plane, raise both arms above your head, bring palms together (interlace or cross fingers), straighten elbows and centre yourself within your personal axis.

3. Take a deep breath and as you exhale, in a straight line within the trajectory of the Coronal Plane bend and stretch arms and upper body over to your right side.

4. Adjust hips, torso, arms and head within the planes, focus your attention on the lower part of your legs, distribute your weight evenly on the soles of your feet and straighten your knees.

5. Lift your breast bone forward, concentrate, focus your eyes on a point in front, breathe naturally and hold the pose for ten seconds.

6. Take a breath and on your exhalation return to the upright position, align yourself within your axis and stretch up.

7. Inhale and on your exhalation stretch over to your left side and repeat the posture exactly the same, stay aware of alignment, weight distribution, breath, focus for ten seconds.

8. Inhale and as you exhale return to your upright position, stretch up and get ready for the Back Bend.

"The sun watches what I do, but the moon knows all my secrets."- *J.M. Wonderland*

1.a. Back Bend (part of Half Moon)

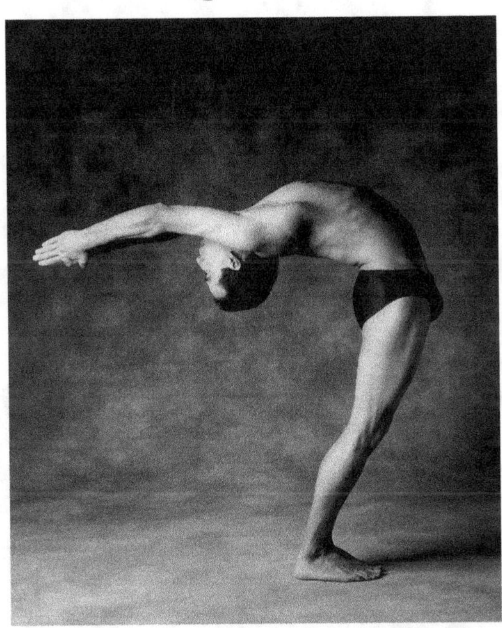

1. Continue from Lateral Half Moon.

2. Keep arms extended above your head, stand within your axis and straighten both elbows. (Students with back issues place hands on the lower back for support)

3. Inhale. On your exhalation extend your head back, following the trajectory of the Sagittal Plane, bend back and slowly stretch arms and torso towards the back as far as you safely can.

4. Lift your breast bone, arch your spine and try to breathe naturally.

5. Focus your attention on the lower part of your legs, distribute your weight evenly on the soles of your feet, and try to straighten both knees.

6. Concentrate, breathe naturally and hold the posture for ten seconds.

7. Inhale. On your exhalation return to your upright position, stand within your axis, stretch up and prepare for Hands to Feet.

"In backbends the outer mind is silenced and the inner mind is made to work."- BKS Iyengar

2. Hands to Feet (Flexion)

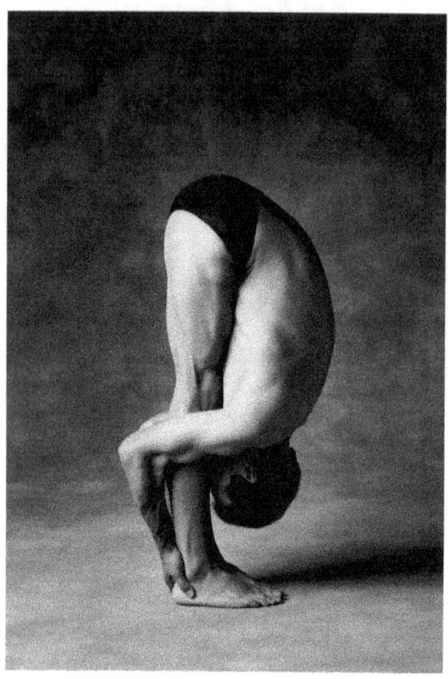

1. Continue from Back Bend.

2. Keeping arms above your head, elbows and knees straight and back as flat as possible, continuing within the trajectory of the Sagittal Plane, slowly and carefully bend and stretch your upper body forward.

3. Once you reach your limit, and can not maintain back and legs straight, slowly bend your knees and relax your body down towards your feet (for students with back issues, place hands on the thighs for support, raise head, flatten back and slowly lower body down).

4. Breathe, then bend knees up and down as if you were doing squats for several times to loosen up your hips.

5. With your knees bent, grab your heels with their respective hands using the "C" grip, bring and squeeze elbows against your calve muscles, and push both shoulders up away from your head.

6. Touch abdomen on your thighs, chest on your knees and face on your shins.

7. Concentrate, breathe naturally and hold the pose for twenty seconds.

8. Inhale. On your exhalation release both heels, extend arms forward, raise head and with flat back return to standing central position.

9. Keep arms above your head, stand within your axis, and stretch up, before bringing arms down to your sides. (Students with back issues place hands on their respective thighs for support when standing up).

10. Stand in the Anatomical Position and relax for a few seconds in preparation for Triangle.

"In forward bends, one uses the outer mind and the inner mind to reach complete silence." - *BKS Iyengar*

3. Triangle

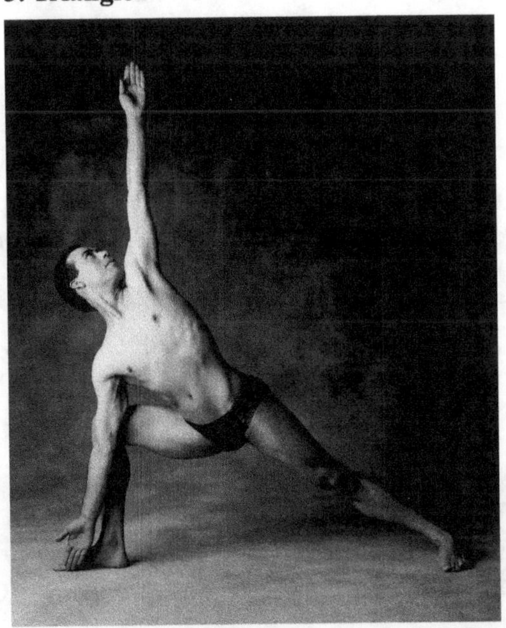

1. Raise your arms above your head, stand in alignment within your axis and stretch up.

2. Inhale. On your exhalation within the trajectory of the Coronal Plane take a wide step to your right side as you lower both arms half way, in line with the Coronal Plane to be parallel with the floor, hand palms facing down.

3. Breathe, centre your body, and within the transverse plane turn your right foot over to your right side, right underneath the right arm.

4. Bend your right knee to create a right angle with your right leg, keep spine straight and centred within your axis.

5. Breathe, tilt your torso over your bent right leg, place elbow against the interior part of your right knee and touch right fingertips on the floor close to your right heel. (students with back issues place elbow on bent leg for support).

6. Raise your left arm straight up, perpendicular to the floor and in line with your right arm.

7. Breathe, centre hips, legs and arms within the Coronal Plane, turn head up and look at your left fingers.
8. Concentrate, breathe naturally and hold the posture for ten seconds.

9. Inhale. On your exhalation turn your face forward, slowly return torso back to your upright position and straighten your right leg.

10. Turn right foot forward and left foot to your left side and repeat posture on the left side exactly the same.

11. Inhale. On your exhalation return back to your upright position, turn feet forward, raise arms above your head, palms together and stretch up.

12. Bring your feet together, lower both arms at your sides and stand in the Anatomical Position in preparation for Standing Separate Leg head to Knee.

"Never be afraid to try. The only angel through which you can approach success is by the "try- angle". You may fail if you try, but shame unto you if you don't try at all. If you fail…rise up and try again and again!"- *Israel More Ayivor*

4. Separate Legs Head to Knee

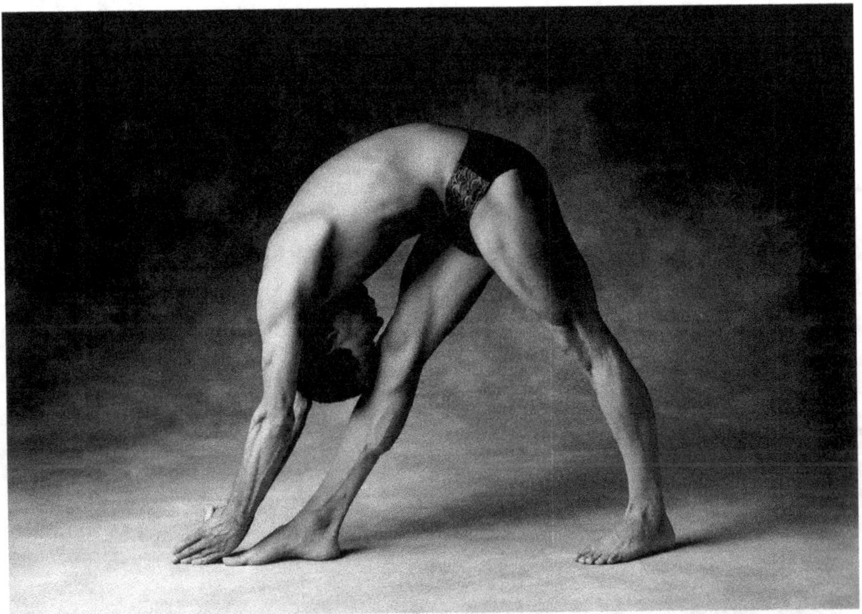

1. Stand in the Anatomical Position, bring both arms above your head, palms together, cross your thumbs and stretch up within your personal axis.

2. Take a breath, and within the trajectory of the Coronal Plane on your exhalation with your right leg take wide step over to your right side (keep arms with palms together above your head).

3. Stretched up, follow the trajectory of the Transverse Plane and slowly turn your right foot, hips, and upper body over to your right side until you are facing your right foot.

4. Breathe, adjust your back left foot in between coronal and sagittal planes and square hips over your right leg.

5. Inhale. On your exhalation tuck your chin down, round your back as you flex your upper body over your right leg, and place sides of your hands on your right foot or floor.

6. Straighten your legs, tuck your chin in and bring your forehead to your right knee as close as you can.

7. Concentrate, breathe naturally and hold the posture for ten seconds.

8. Inhale. On your exhalation raise your head, extend arms over your right leg, look up, flatten your back and return to standing position, still facing your right foot. (students with back issues place hands on the right thigh for support when standing up).

9. Breathe, turn right foot, torso, head and arms forward, then turn left foot, hips and upper body over to your left side, and repeat the pose exactly the same and hold it for ten seconds.

10. Inhale. On your exhalation return to standing position, turn left foot and upper body forward, bring feet together, slowly lower both arms to your sides, and stand in the Anatomical Position to prepare for Awkward.

"More stretching less stressing."- **myoga**

5. Awkward (three parts)

PART ONE

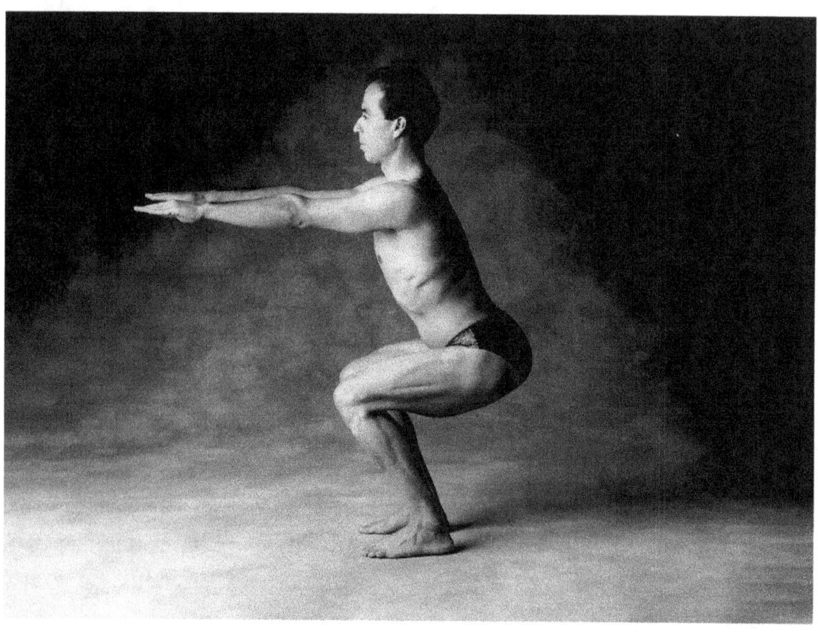

1. Stand tall in the Anatomical Position and breathe.

2. Within the trajectory of the coronal plane separate feet shoulder width apart, and stand tall.

3. Follow the trajectory of the sagittal plane, straighten and raise both arms

up until they are parallel to the floor, in line with your feet and keep fingers together and palms facing down.

4. Breathe, push buttocks slightly back, extend and raise your breast bone forward and up.

5. Slowly bend knees as much as you can or until the back of your thighs are parallel to the floor.

6. Concentrate, breathe naturally and hold the pose for ten seconds.

7. Inhale. On your exhalation, slowly return to standing, starting position and get ready for the second part.
"The days you are most uncomfortable are the days you learn the most about yourself."- **Therandomvibes**

PART TWO

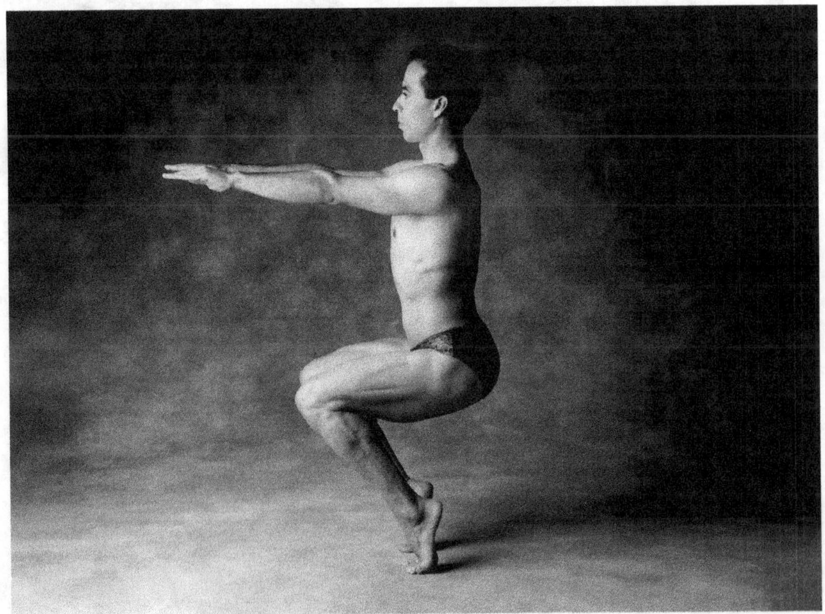

1. Continue from first part of Awkward.

2. Keep feet shoulder width apart and arms parallel to the floor, and breathe.

3. Concentrate on one point in front on the floor, and slowly stand on your toes as high as can.

4. Breathe, push your buttocks slightly back, extend and raise breast bone forward and on your tiptoes bend both knees as much as you can or until the back of your legs are parallel to the floor and arms parallel to your legs.

5. Extend and straighten your spine as much as possible focus, and breathe as naturally as you can.

6. Concentrate, look for stillness within the posture and hold it for ten seconds.

7. Inhale. On your exhalation stand up, lower your heels and get ready for the third part.

"Whatever makes you uncomfortable is your biggest opportunity for growth."-Bryant McGull

PART THREE

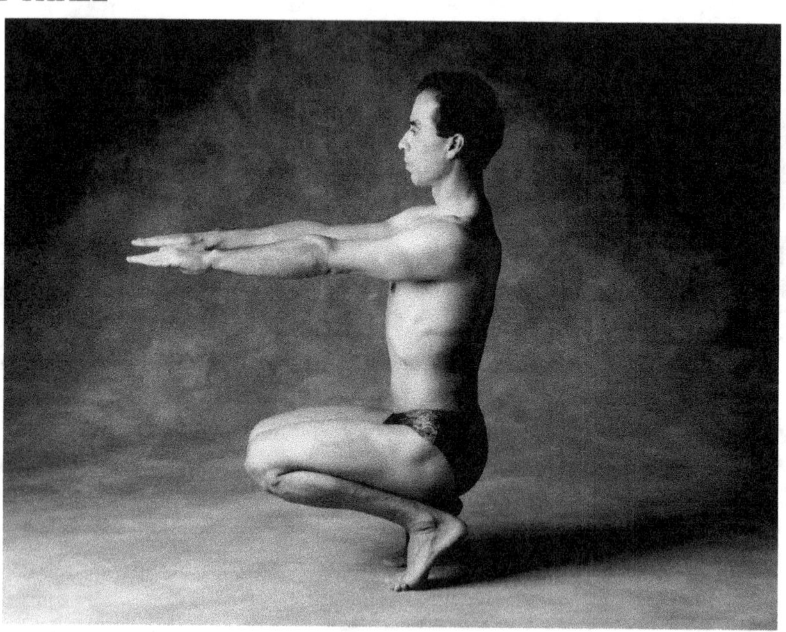

1. With arms parallel to the floor stand tall, raise your heels slightly off the floor, balance on the balls of your feet and bring knees together.

2. Breathe, then push your buttocks back and slowly lower yourself until your butt barely touches on your heels.

3. Keeping your arm muscles firm, bring knees parallel with the floor and squeeze your inner thighs together.

4. Straighten and keep your spine perpendicular to the floor, your body should form a perfect square with torso, thighs and arms.

5. Concentrate, breathe naturally and hold the pose for twenty seconds.

6. Inhale. On your exhalation, separate knees, stand up, lower heels to the floor, lower arms and stand in the Anatomical Position in preparation for Eagle.

"Life begins at the end of your comfort zone."- *Neale Donald Walsch*

6. Eagle (Right & Left Sides)

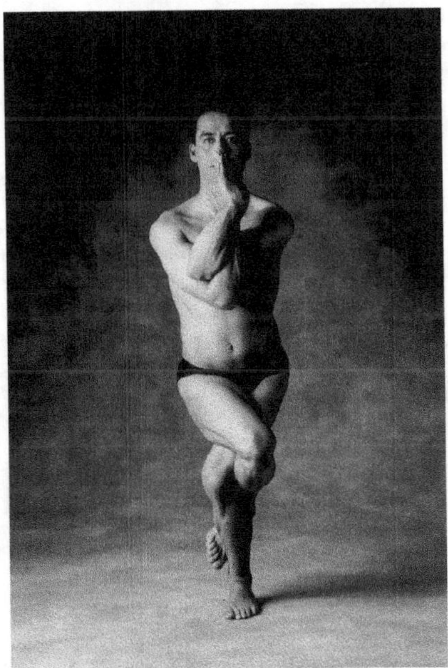 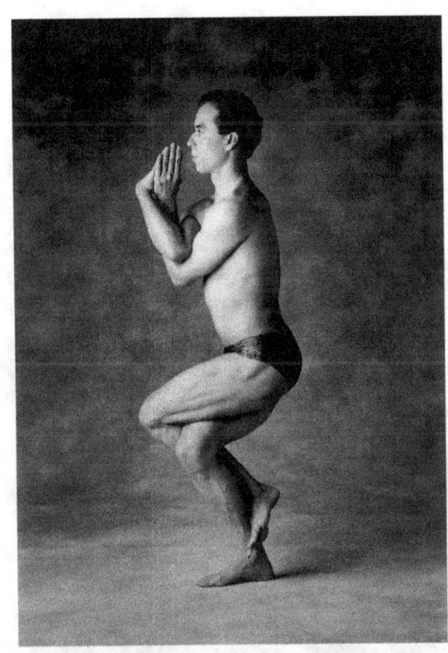

1. Stand tall in Anatomical Position and breathe.

2. Raise both arms above your head to form a big"V" within the Coronal Plane.

3. Lean slightly forward, bring and cross your right arm under the left arm, clasp hands together and straighten your back.

4. Centre your elbows in front of your chest and thumbs in front of your face.
5. Breathe, and slowly take a small step forward with your left foot, stick and push your buttocks slightly back, then bend both knees about six inches.

6. Shift your weight onto your front left leg and balance.

7. Raise your right knee straight up towards your chest and then, slowly cross your right leg over your upper left thigh and bring your right foot behind your standing left ankle.

8. Sink deeper into standing leg, level your shoulders and hips, and align elbows and knees with the Sagittal Plane.

9. Concentrate, breathe naturally and hold the posture for twenty seconds.

10. Inhale. On your exhalation undo the pose and return to Anatomical Position in preparation for the left side.

11. Raise your arms up above your head and repeat the posture on the left side exactly the same as in the right side.

12. Once finished, stand in the Anatomical Position in preparation for Standing Head to Knee "The Eagle does not escape the storm.

The Eagle simply uses the storm to lift higher. It spreads its mighty wings and rises on the winds that bring the storm." - *Jack White*

7. Standing Head to Knee (Right & Left Sides)

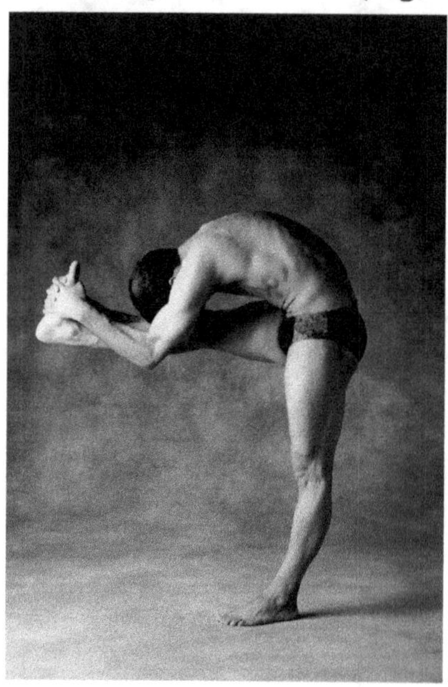

1. Stand tall in Anatomical Position, and breathe.

2. Follow the trajectory of the Sagittal Plane and with your left foot take a small step forward.

3. Shift your weight onto your front left leg and with your body straight up, raise right knee up towards your chest as high as you can.

4. Keep you right knee high up, bend forward, interlace fingers, and grab the ball of your right foot firmly, and place thumbs on top of your foot.

5. Breathe, align your body, and slowly, following the Sagittal Plane extend your right leg forward until it is parallel to the floor, forming a right angle with standing left leg.

6. Bring elbows in and down toward your right calf muscle, then lower your torso as close as you can to your upper leg.

7. If possible, tuck chin into your chest and and bring your forehead to your knee.

8. Concentrate, breathe naturally and hold the pose for twenty seconds.

9. Inhale. On your exhalation slowly raise your body up, lower your upper leg to undo the pose and return to the Anatomical Position and prepare for the left side.

10. Breathe, take a step forward with your right foot and repeat the posture on the left side exactly the same as the right side to completion.

11. Stand tall in Anatomical Position to prepare for Standing Bow.

"Balance in not something you find, it's something you create."- *Jana Kingsford*

8. Standing Bow (Right & Left Sides)

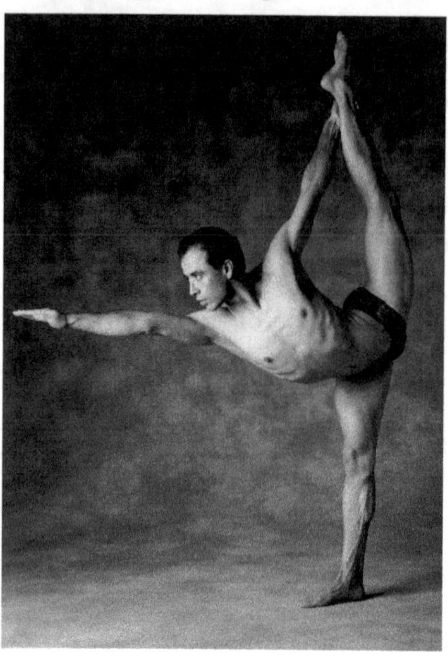

1. Stand tall in Anatomical Position and breathe.

2. With your left foot take a small step forward within the Sagittal Plane, transfer your weight onto it and breathe.

3. Extend your right arm behind you with elbow and palm facing away from the body.

4. Lift your right foot back towards your right buttock and from the inside of your leg, with your right hand grab your foot firmly.

5. Keep your upper right knee close to your standing left leg, centre your hips and raise your left arm as high as you can in front of your body with fingers together and palm facing down.

6. Inhale. On your exhalation following the Sagittal Plane and with your head held high, tilt your upper body forward and at the same time with pointed toes raise your right leg up towards the ceiling.

7. Lower your torso forward, keep your right hip facing down, arch your spine, hold your head up, and lift your right leg as high as you can without twisting.

8. Concentrate, breathe naturally and hold the posture for ten seconds.

9. Inhale. On your exhalation undo the pose, return to the Anatomical Position and prepare for the left side.

10. Take a step forward with your right foot, raise your left leg back and repeat the posture on the left side exactly the same.

11. After completing the posture return to the Anatomical Position and prepare for Balancing Stick.

"Life is a balance between holding on and letting go."- *Rumi*

9. Balancing Stick (Right & Left Sides)

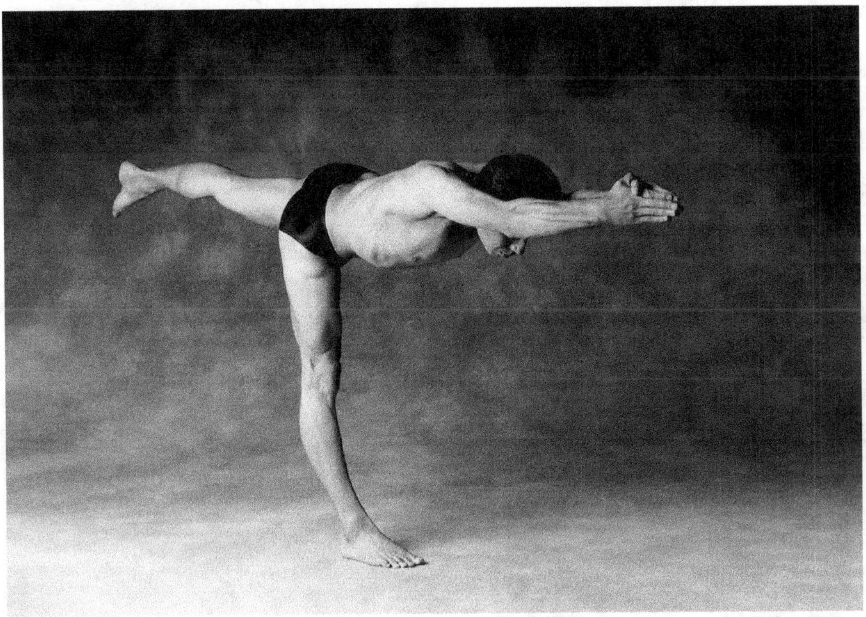

1. Stand tall in the Anatomical Position and breathe.

2. Within the coronal plane, raise both arms above your head, palms together, cross your thumbs and stretch up towards the ceiling, along your personal axis.

3. With your right foot take a step forward, shift your weight onto it and breathe.

4. Following the Sagittal Plane, with a flat back and arms above your head, slowly tilt your upper body forward and down and at the same time lift your back left leg up until your entire body from tiptoes to fingertips is parallel to the floor.

5. Level your hips, straighten both legs and stretch upper body forward, and upper left leg back.

6. Concentrate, breathe naturally and hold the posture for ten seconds.

7. Inhale. On your exhalation return to starting position, keep arms above your head and prepare for the left side.

8. Breathe, step forward with your left foot, shift your weight onto it and repeat pose on the left side exactly the same, after completion return to the Anatomical Position to prepare for Splits in the Air.

"The secret to life is finding the right balance to everything you do."- *Unknown*

10. Splits in the Air (Right & Left Sides)

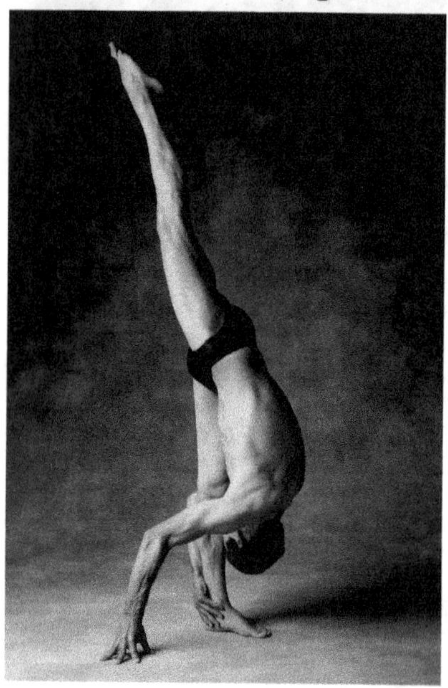

1. Stand tall in the Anatomical Position, and breathe.

2. Raise both arms above your head, palms together and stretch up along the your axis.

3. Inhale. On your exhalation, with your right foot take a step forward and shift your weight on to it.

4. Following the sagittal plane and in one continuous motion tilt your upper

body forward and down as you slowly raise your left leg up towards the ceiling, place both hands on the floor, make sure your foot is in between them.

5. Inhale. On your exhalation, with your right hand grab your standing right ankle and press elbow against your right calf muscle.

6. Use your left hand for support, roll your right hip down until it is properly aligned with the planes and straighten your standing leg before lifting upper leg even higher.

7. Concentrate, breathe naturally and hold the posture for ten seconds.

8. Inhale. On your exhalation release your ankle, look forward and with a flat back return your upper body up to standing starting position as you lower your left leg, place your left foot on the floor, and stand tall.

9. Keep your arms above head, with your left foot take a step forward and repeat the posture on the left side exactly the same.

10. Breathe, complete pose on the left side, return to standing position, lower arms, stand in Anatomical Position and prepare for Separate Leg Stretching.

"Two things I'm trying to work on are openness and flexibility."- *Lili Taylor*

11. Separate Leg Stretching

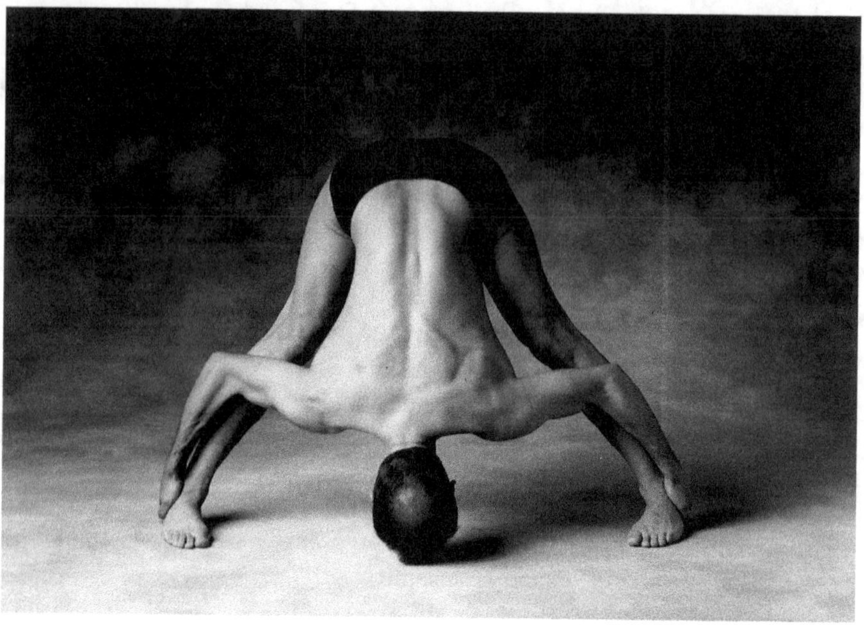

1. Stand tall in the Anatomical Position and breathe.

2. Following the Coronal Plane raise both arms above your head, palms together and stretch up along your axis.
3. Inhale. On your exhalation within the sagittal plane, take a wide step to your right side, lower arms parallel to floor with palms facing down.

4. Take a breath and as you exhale, with a flat back slowly, bring your upper body forward and down as much as you can, and grab heels with their respective hands.

5. Straighten your legs, ground your feet, straighten your back, and raise your head.

6. Bend and keep elbows close to your lower legs and if possible touch your forehead on floor.

7. Concentrate, breathe naturally and hold the pose for twenty seconds.

8. Inhale. On your exhalation release heels, raise head, extend arms sideways and with a flat back stand up, return to your standing, starting position and bring arms above your head.

9. Inhale. On your exhalation bring feet together, lower arms to your sides,

stand in the Anatomical Position and prepare for Tree Pose.

"You must always be able to predict what's next and then the flexibility to evolve."- *Marc Benioff*

12. Tree (Right & Left Sides)

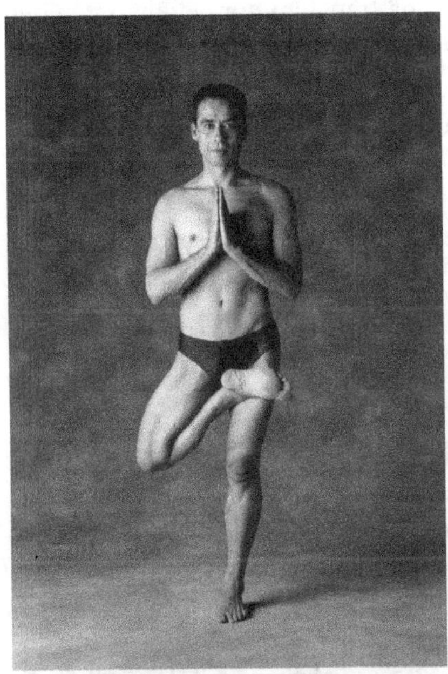

1. Stand tall in the Anatomical Position and breathe.

2. Take a small step forward with your left foot and transfer your weight onto your front left leg.

3. Following the Sagittal Plane raise your right knee up towards your abdomen, bend upper body slightly forward and with both hands grab your right foot, pull it up towards your abdomen and place it as high as possible on your upper left thigh.

4. Straighten your body, push your right knee down and back and if your foot stays on your thigh by itself bring both hands in front of your chest in a praying position, otherwise keep holding it with your left hand and bring your right hand up to your chest.

5. Stand tall along your axis, lift chest and breast bone forward and relax your shoulders.

6. Concentrate, breathe naturally and hold the posture for ten seconds.

7. Inhale. On your exhalation slowly with help of your hands lower your right foot to the floor, stand in the Anatomical Position and preparation for the left side.

8. Take a small step forward with your right foot, transfer your weight onto your front leg and repeat the posture on the left side exactly the same.

9. Inhale. On your exhalation undo the left side, stand in the Anatomical Position and prepare for Finger Stand.

"The trees that are slow to grow bear the best fruit". - *Unknown*

13. Corpose Pose (Savasana)

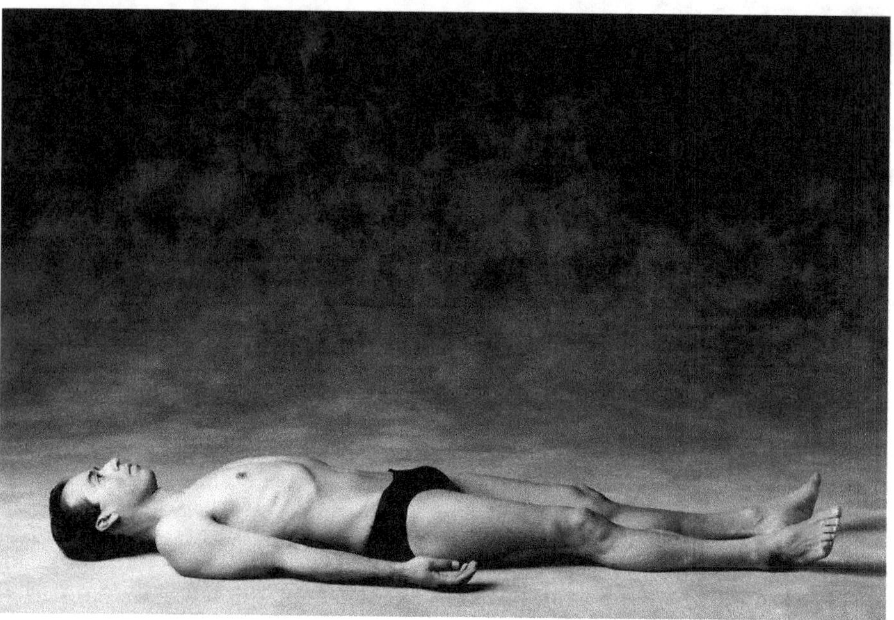

1. Lie down on your mat with face up, spine and legs aligned and heels slightly apart.

2. Breathe, relax body from the inside out starting with your spine, skeleton, joints, muscles and skin.

3. Focus your attention on your cerebral cortex, cerebellum, brainstem, spinal cord and finally on your heart and lungs.

4. Think positive thoughts, look for inner peace and create a positive self image.
5. Concentrate, breathe naturally and relax for twenty seconds in preparation for Wind Removing pose.

"Your mind will answer most questions if you learn to relax and wait for the answer."- *William S. Burroughs*

14. Wind Relieving (three parts)

PART ONE

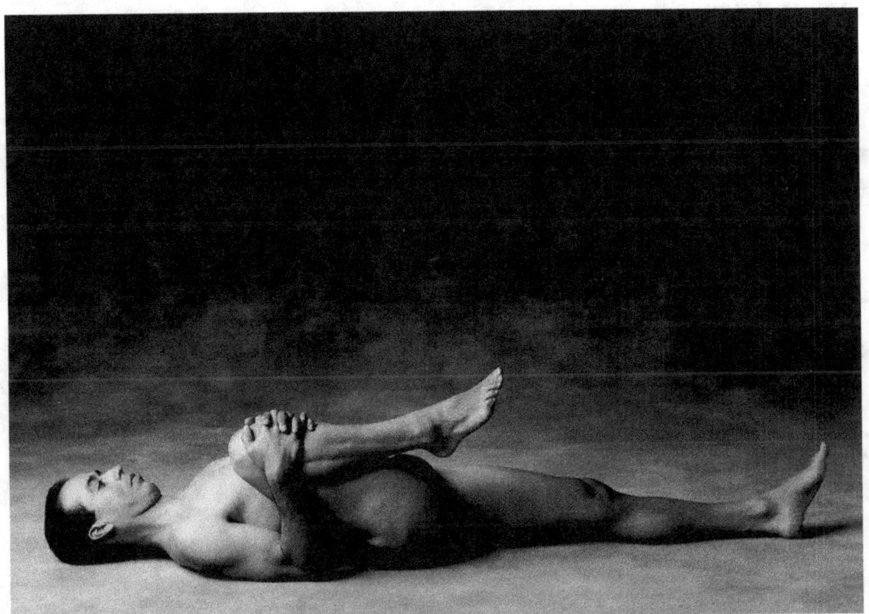

1. At the end of Savasana, following the Sagittal Plane, raise your right knee up to your chest, interlace your fingers and grab your leg two inches below knee.

2. Breathe and pull your knee as close as possible to your right shoulder.
3. Straighten your left leg, keep head on floor, tuck your chin in and bring elbows close to your rib cage.

4. Concentrate, breathe naturally and hold posture for ten seconds.

5. Inhale. On your exhalation undo hands, lower your right leg to floor and get ready for left side.

"Be like the lotus: trust in the light; grow through the dirt; believe in new beginnings." - *aimhappy.com*

PART TWO

1. Inhale. On your exhalation raise your left leg to your chest and repeat pose exactly the same.

2. After completing the posture, lower your left leg to floor and get ready for part three.

"Throw caution to the wind and just do it."- *Carrie Underwood*

PART THREE

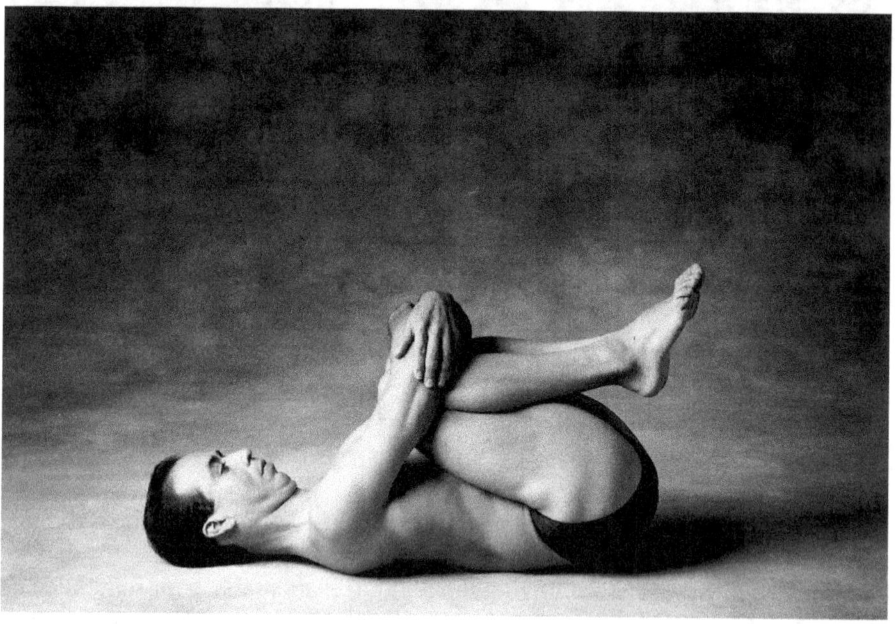

1. Inhale. On your exhalation within the sagittal plane bring both knees up to your chest, cross arms over your legs and grab opposite elbows with their respective hands.

2. Breathe, tuck chin in, flatten spine and push hips down.

3. Keep legs together, move shoulders away from your head and flatten rib cage on the floor.

4. Concentrate, breathe and hold pose for twenty seconds.

5. Inhale. On your exhalation release elbows and undo pose.

6. Relax in Savasana for ten seconds in preparation for the Sit-up.

"Anger is a wind which blows out the lamp of the mind."- *Robert Green*

Sit-up

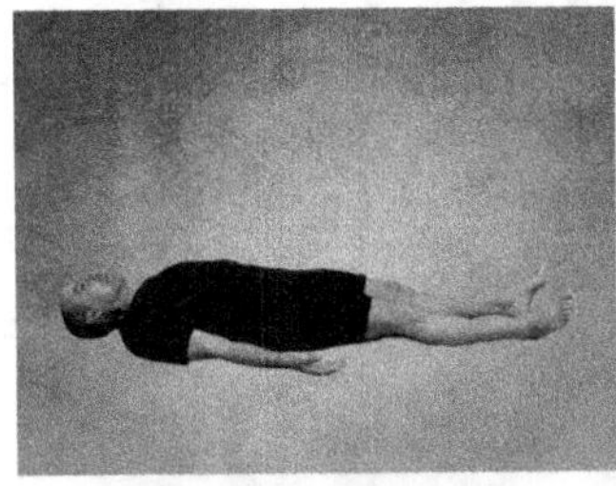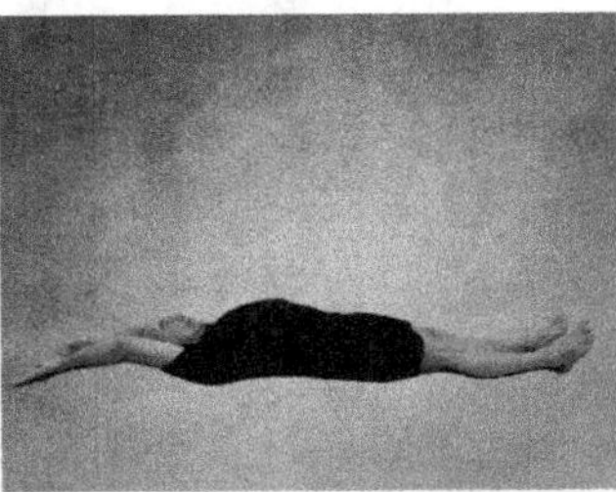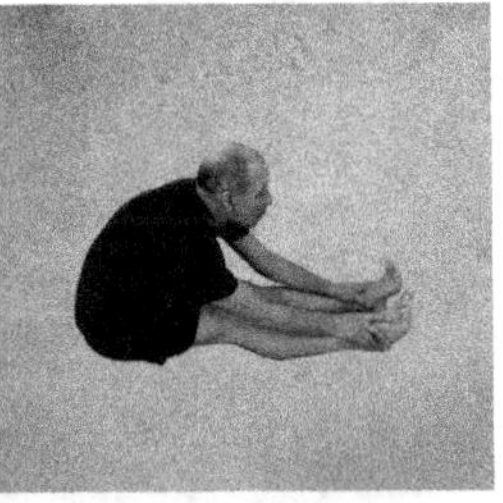

1. In Savasana, become aware of your own weight, bring feet together and straighten both legs.

2. Raise both arms above your head, keep palms facing up and inhale.

3. Exhale completely and at the base of exhalation with one motion sit up, dive forward over your legs and touch toes with your hands.

4. Breathe, turn around, lay face down on the mat and get ready for the Cobra pose.

"It is easy to sit up and take notice, what is difficult is getting up and taking action."- *Honore de Balzac*

15. Cobra

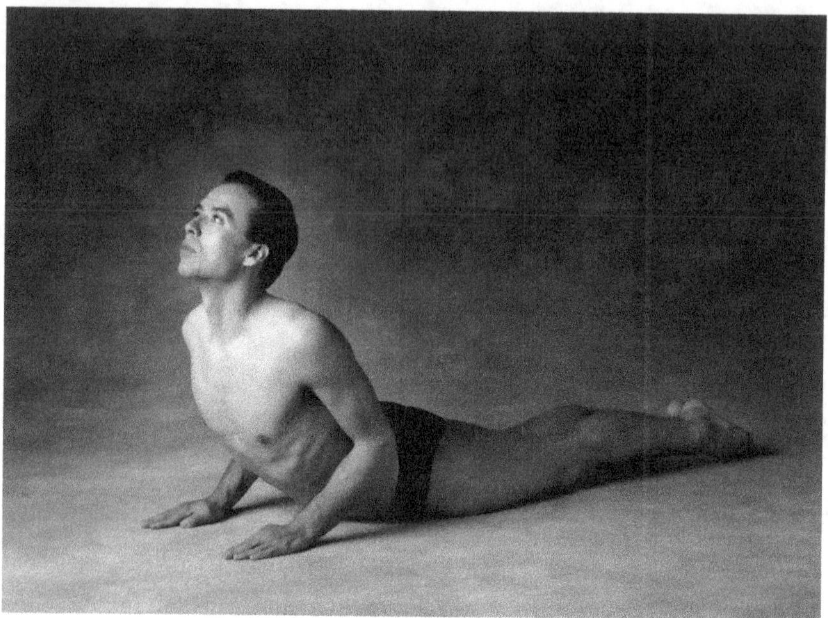

1. Laying face down on your mat along the Sagittal Plane, place hand palms flat on the floor under your chest, keep fingers together and inline with contour of your shoulders.

2. Bring face forward, place chin on the floor, press elbows against your rib cage, bring legs together, point your toes back, and breathe.

3. On your inhalation, mainly using back and abdominal muscle strength raise your torso off the floor to a forty-five degree angle or until your bellybutton barely touches the floor.

4. Tighten your legs and buttock's muscles for support, arch your back and push your breast bone forward.

5. Concentrate, breathe naturally and hold posture for twenty seconds.

6. Inhale. On your exhalation lower your body, turn face to one side, bring arms down at your sides and relax in Savasana for ten seconds in preparation for Locust pose.

"Cobras are magical. They can stand up on just energy alone."- *Paz de la Huerta*

16. Locust (three parts)

PART ONE

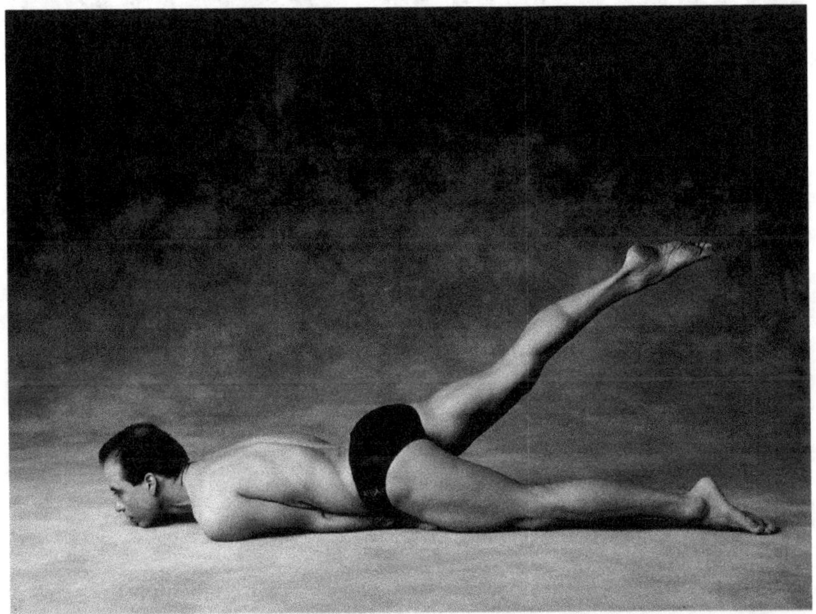

1. Stay face down on your mat, be conscious of your breath, align yourself within the Sagittal Plane and breathe.
2. Bring both arms under your body, place elbows under your abdomen, hands close to each other under your thighs with palms facing down, fingers slightly separate and breathe.

3. Place your chin on the floor, and on your exhalation extend and lift your right leg up to a forty-five degree angle from the floor.

4. Concentrate, breathe naturally and hold the posture for ten seconds.

5. Inhale. On your exhalation lower your right leg and prepare for the left side.

"Neglect of yoga practice is the locust which devours the strength of the body."-
T Sanchez

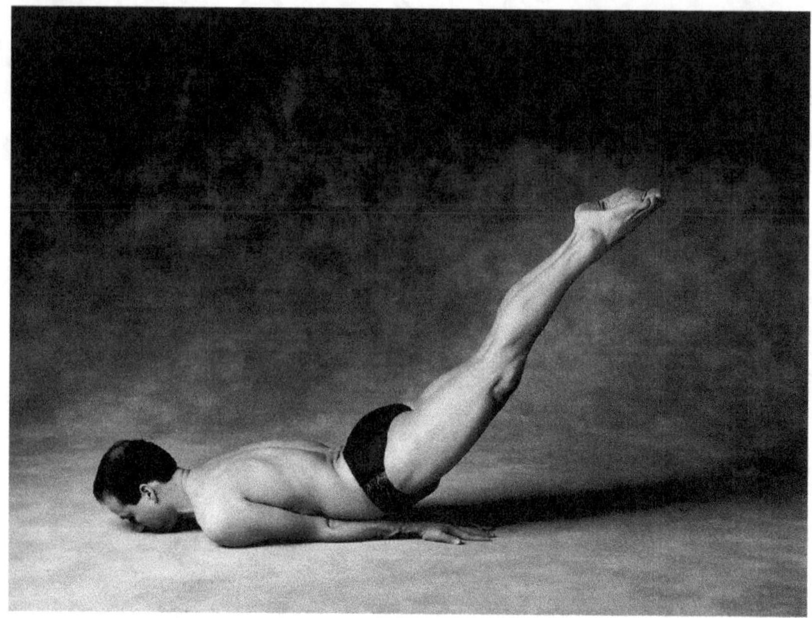

1. Inhale. On your exhalation raise your left leg and repeat the pose exactly the same.

2. Inhale. On your exhalation lower your left leg and prepare for third part.

"Locust have leg muscles that are about 1000 times more powerful than an equal wight of human muscle."- *Unknown*

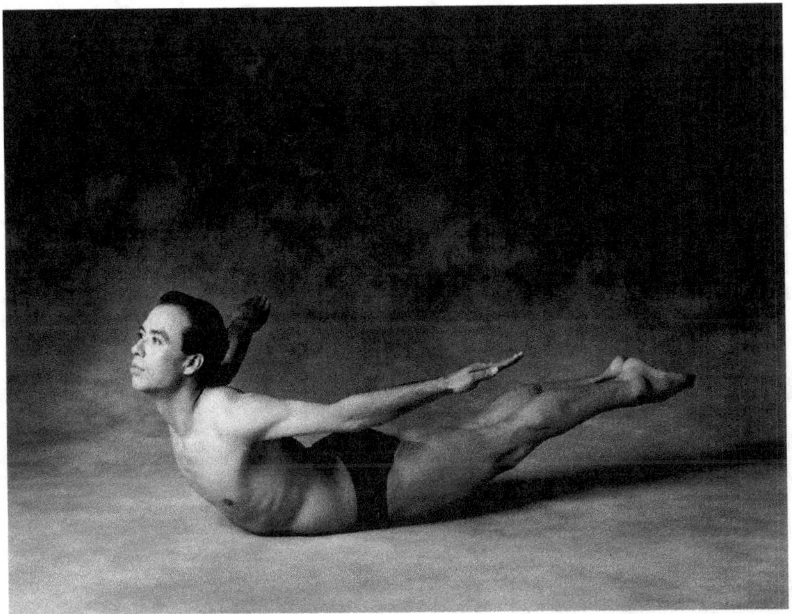

1. Place your mouth on the floor, push shoulders back and down away from your head.

2. Inhale. On your exhalation press fingertips on the floor and together raise both legs as high as you can.

3. Take shallow breaths, straighten both knees, point toes and bring feet closer together.

4. Concentrate, take shallow breaths and hold pose for ten seconds.

5. On your exhalation, lower your legs to the floor, pull arms out from under your body, turn your face to one side and relax in Savasana for ten seconds in preparation for Full Locust.

"There is no force equal to that of a determined mind."- *imgur*

17. Full Locust

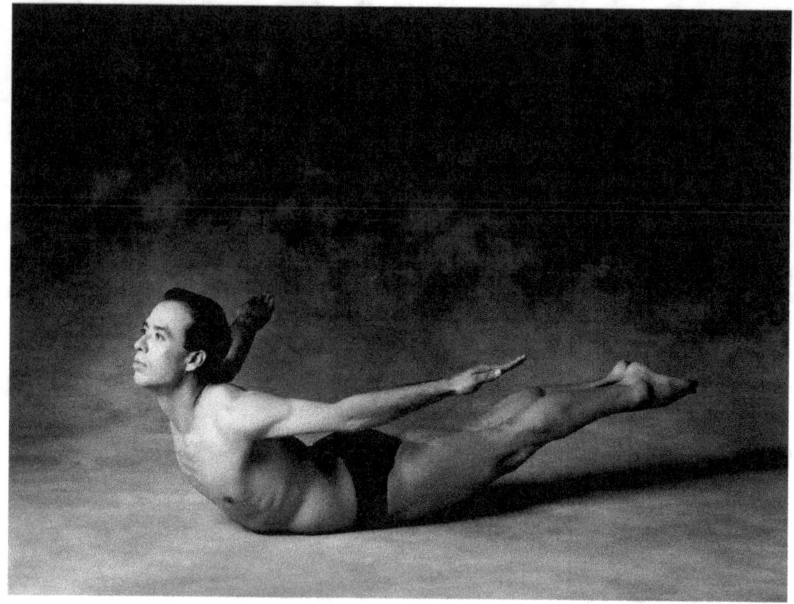

1. Stay alert, turn your face forward, place your chin on the mat, and breathe.

2. Within the Transverse Plane, move arms away from your torso to a forty-five degree angle from your spine with palms facing down.

3. Bring legs together, point your toes back and extend your spine.

4. On your inhalation, at the same time raise your upper body and legs off the floor as high as can.

5. Straighten your legs, bring arms back and up to compress your shoulder blades together, and breathe.

6. Push your breast bone forward, and open your chest as you raise your upper body higher.

7. Concentrate, breathe naturally and hold the posture for ten seconds.

8. On your exhalation lower your body down, turn your face to one side and relax in Savasana for ten seconds in preparation for Bow.

"I will restore to you the years that the swarming locust has eaten."- *Joel 2:25*

18. Bow

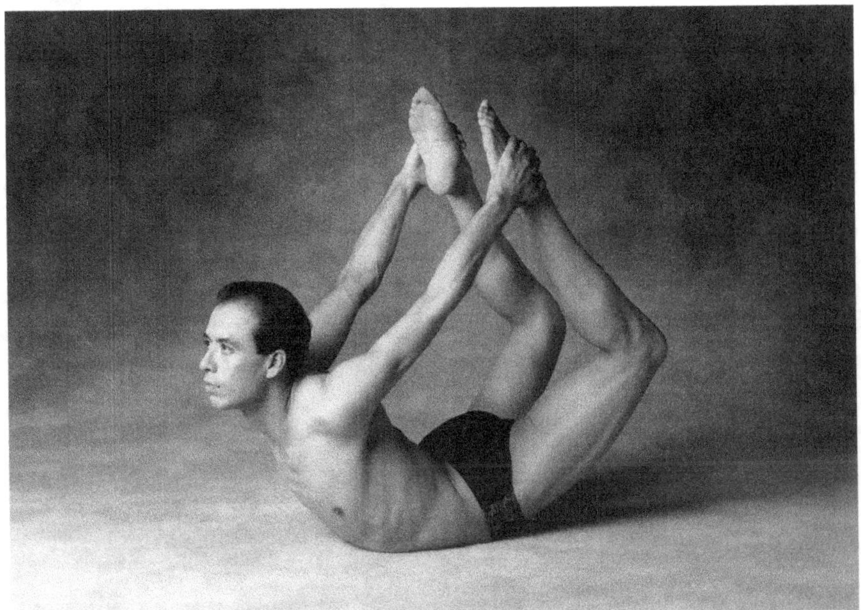

1. Be conscious of your breath and turn your face forward, and breathe.

2. Following the trajectory of the Sagittal Plane, bend both knees and bring feet straight up towards your buttock, and grab them with their respective hands.

3. Separate knees and feet shoulder width apart, bring shoulder blades close to each other, extend head forward and up, and breathe.

4. On your inhalation, using the strength of your legs raise your upper body and thighs off floor as high as high as you can.

5. Maintain the distance in between your legs, look up, open your chest and slightly roll back towards your lower abdomen.

6. Concentrate, breathe naturally and hold the posture for twenty seconds.

7. Inhale. On your exhalation lower body down, turn face to one side, palms up and relax in Savasana for ten seconds in preparation for Half Tortoise.

"When in doubt put a bow on it."- *TatToes*

19. Half Tortoise

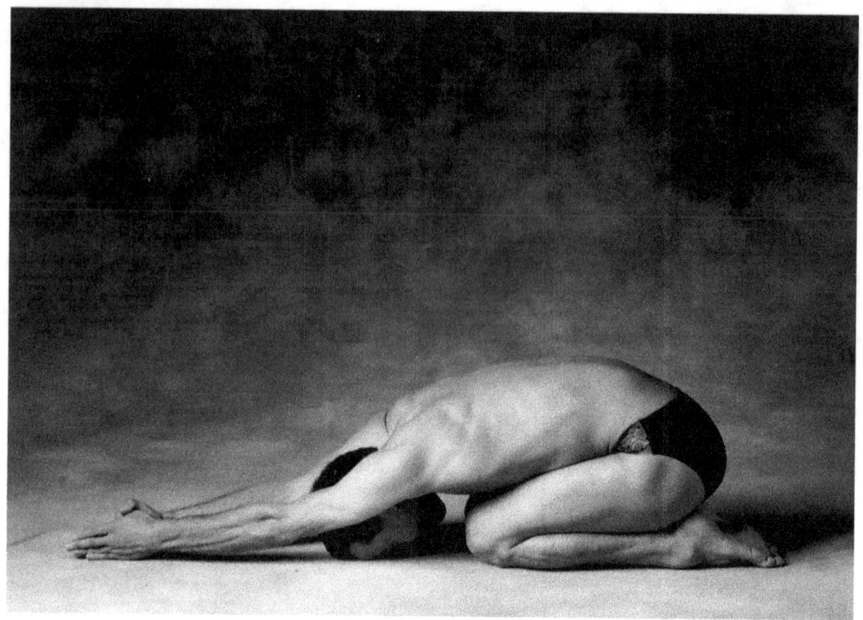

1. Kneel down Japanese style, straighten your spine, centre your head and breathe.

2. Follow the trajectory of the Coronal Plane, raise both arms above your head, palms together and centre your upper body and arms with your axis.

3. Follow the trajectory of the Sagittal Plane, and on your exhalation with your head held high, back flat, and arms fully extended bring your upper body over your bent legs, placing abdomen on your thighs, chest on your knees and forehead and side of your hands on the floor.

4. Keep your buttocks as close as possible to your heels, elbows in the air and stretch forward.
5. Concentrate, keep eyes open, breathe naturally and hold posture for twenty seconds.

6. Take a breath, and with flat back and arms fully extended return back to starting sitting position.

7. Inhale. On your exhalation lower your arms, lay down on your back and relax in Savasana for ten seconds preparation for Sit-up and Camel Pose.

"Slow and steady wins the race."- *Aesop's Fables*

Sit-up

1. In Savasana, become aware of your own weight, bring feet together and straighten both legs.

2. Raise both arms above your head shoulder width apart, keep palms facing up and inhale.

3. Exhale completely and at the base of exhalation with one motion sit up, dive forward over your legs and touch toes with your hands.

4. Turn around and stand up on your knees for Camel.

"Worry less, smile more. Don't regret, just learn and grow."- *Buddha Groove*

20. Camel

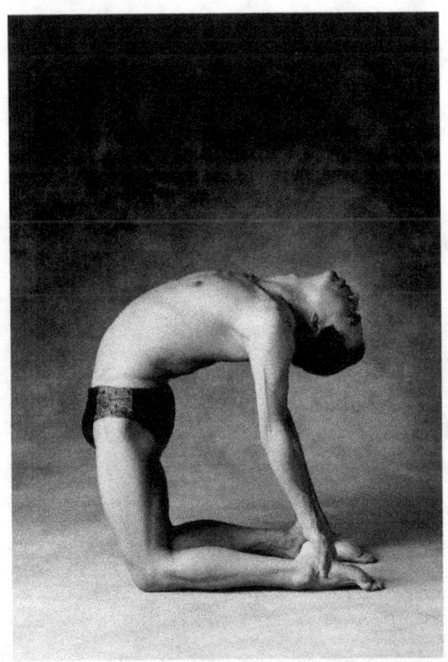

1. Stand on your knees, shoulder width apart and breathe.

2. Place your hands on your lower back, fingertips pointing down towards the floor, raise your breast bone up , and extend your head.

3. Following the Sagittal Plane, extend and bend your upper body back, push hips slightly forward and bring your shoulder blades together.

4. Breathe and slowly lower your hands down to their respective heels one at

the time, and grab them firmly.

5. Push your thighs and hips forward, lift your chest up, move both shoulders away from your head, and extend your head back.

6. Concentrate, breathe naturally and the hold the posture for twenty seconds.

7. Inhale. On your exhalation bring hands one at the time to your lower back and return to starting kneeling position.

8. Relax in Savasana for ten seconds in preparation for the Sit-up and Rabbit Pose.

"Life is like a camel: you can make it do anything except back up." - *Marcelene Cox*

Sit-up
1. In Savasana, become aware of your own weight, bring feet together and straighten both legs.

2. Raise arms above your head, keep palms facing up and inhale.

3. Exhale completely and at the base of exhalation with one motion sit up, dive forward over your legs and touch toes with your hands.

4. Turn around, kneel down with knees and feet together.

"I don't count my sit-ups; I only start counting when it starts burning because they're the only ones that count."- *Muhammad Ali*

21. Rabbit

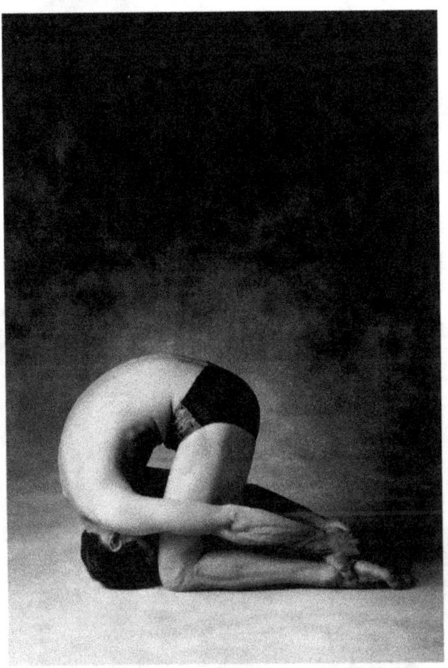

1. Kneel down Japanese style, and breathe.

2. Lean forward, tuck your chin into your chest, bring forehead close to your knees, and grab both heels with respective hands firmly.

3. Inhale. On your exhalation touch your forehead to your knees, top of your head lightly touching on the floor and lift your buttocks off your heels.

4. Keep most of your weight on your arms as you roll forward, and very little on your head.

5. Bring heels together, squeeze legs tightly with your arms, lift shoulders away from your head and pull your abdominal muscles in.

6. Concentrate, breathe naturally, and hold the pose for twenty seconds.

7. Inhale. On your exhalation undo the pose, sit up straight.

8. Turn around, lay down on your back and relax in Savasana for twenty seconds to prepare for the Sit-up before Head to Knee pose.

"Is not always necessary to hop in the direction other bunnies expect." - Bunny Buddhism

Sit-up

1. In Savasana, become aware of your own weight, bring feet together and straighten both legs.

2. Raise arms above your head, keep palms facing up and inhale.

3. Exhale completely and at the base of exhalation with one motion sit up, dive forward over your legs and touch toes with your hands.

4. Turn around, sit on the mat with feet straight forward.

"Fit is not a destination. It's a way of life."- *Crossrope*

22. Head to Knee

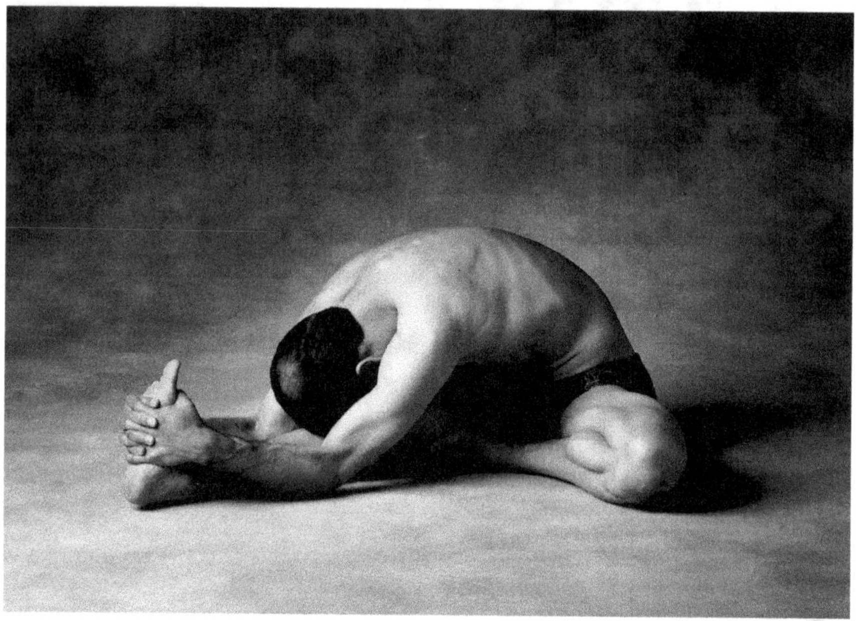

1. Sit with legs extended forward along the sagittal plane, and breathe.

2. Follow the trajectory of the Transverse Plane, and move your right leg to a forty-five degree over to your right side.

3. Breathe, bend your left leg, placing left foot against your inner right thigh with heel as close as possible to your perineum.

4. Raise both arms above your head, interlace your fingers, and turn upper body over to your extended right leg.

5. Take a breath, and on your exhalation bend your upper body over your right leg, and with interlaced fingers grab your right foot firmly.

6. Tuck your chin into your chest, bend your elbows down close to your calf muscle, round your spine, touch your forehead to your right knee and elbows to the floor.

7. Concentrate, breathe naturally, and hold posture for ten seconds.

8. Take a breath, and on your exhalation let go of your foot and return to sitting position.

9. Unbend and extend your left leg over to your left side, bend your right leg, place. Your right foot on the inside of your right thigh repeat the pose exactly the same, and hold for ten seconds.

10. After completion, undo pose, extend both legs forward, bring feet together, lay back and prepare for a quick sit-up before doing the Stretching posture.

"There is nothing in this world that can trouble you as much as your own thoughts."

Sit-up
1. In Savasana, become aware of your own weight, bring feet together and straighten both legs.

2. Raise both arms above your head, keep palms facing up and inhale.

3. Exhale completely and at the base of exhalation with one motion sit up, dive forward over your legs and touch toes with your hands.
"Even if you're on the right track, you'll get run over if you just sit there."- *Will Rogers*

23. Stretching

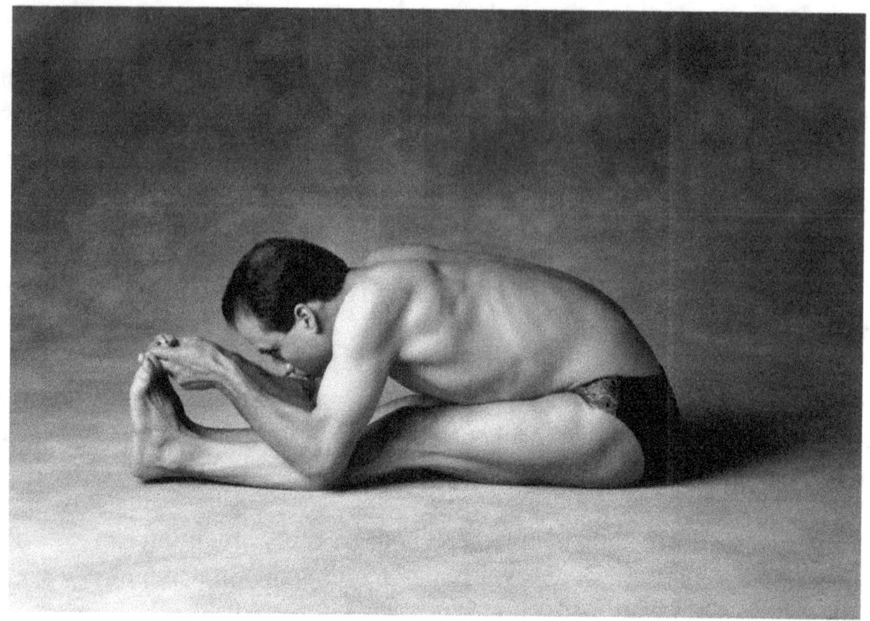

1. This pose is a continuation of Head to knee.

2. Keeping legs extended forward and feet together within the Sagittal Plane, with index and middle fingers grab their respective big toes.

3. Breathe, flatten your back, hold your head up and pull on your toes as you stretch over your legs.

4. Bend your elbows, place them close to your legs, look forward, and reach forward with your head to try to touch forehead to your toes.

5. Concentrate, breathe naturally and hold the posture for twenty seconds.

6. Inhale. On your exhalation undo the pose and prepare for Separate Leg Stretching.

"By stretching yourself beyond your perceived level of confidence you accelerate your development of competence." - *Michael J. Gelb*

23.a. Separate Legs Stretching

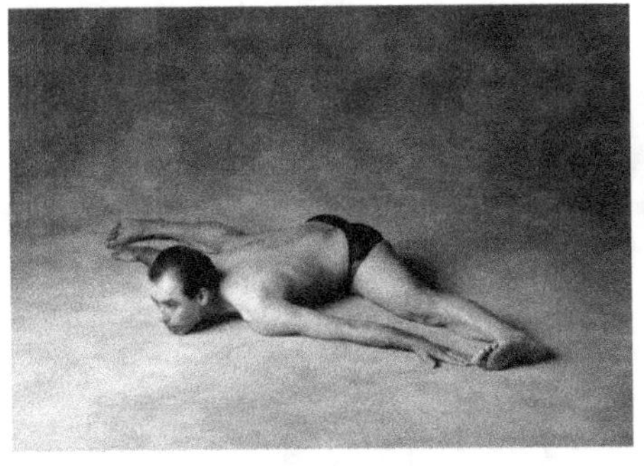 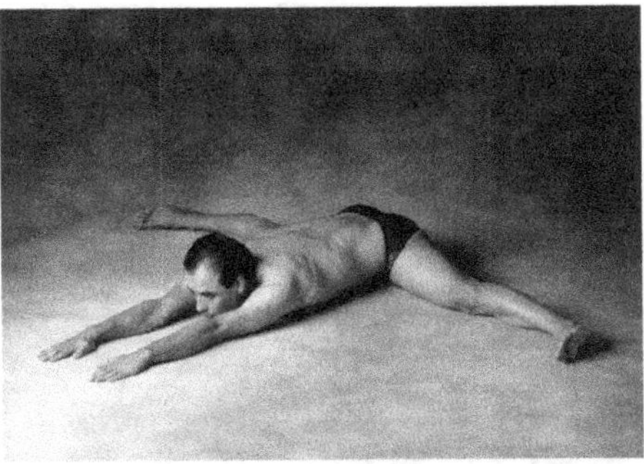

1. Continue from Stretching.

2. Straighten your upper body, and within the transverse plane, separate both legs as much as you can, and breathe.

3. Flex your feet, extend your arms out towards them, and with their respective hands grab your big toes, and roll legs and feet forward as much as you can.

4. Breathe, let go of your toes, extend both arms forward in between your feet, place hand palms on the floor shoulder width apart, hold your head up, and with a flat back walk hands forward as much as you can. (Your goal is to eventually place chest and abdomen flat on the floor.)

5. Concentrate, breathe naturally and hold pose for ten seconds.

6. Inhale. On your exhalation walk hands back, undo pose and prepare for Upward Stretching.

"In a person's career, well, if you're process-oriented and not totally outcome-oriented, then you're more likely to be successful. I often say pursue excellence, ignore success. Success is a by-product of excellence." - *Deepak Chopra*

24. Upward Stretching

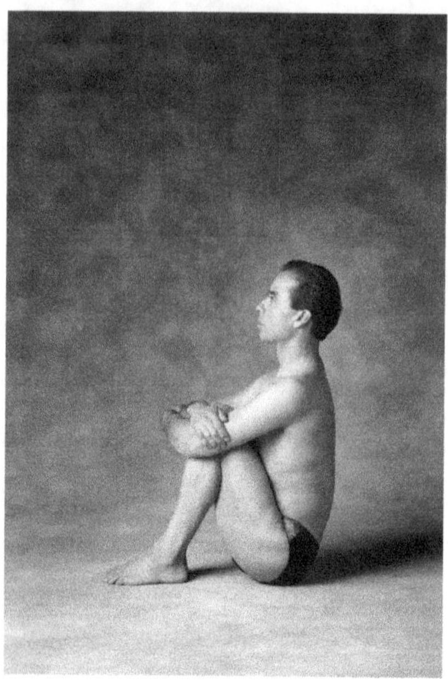

1. Continue from Separate Leg Stretching.

2. Breathe and bring legs together within the Sagittal Plane.

3. Bring both knees into your chest, keep feet flat on floor, wrap arms around your legs and grab the opposite elbows with your hands.

4. Adjust your body, straighten your spine, pull your shoulders down and hold your head up.

5. Concentrate, breathe naturally and hold posture for ten seconds.

6. Inhale. On your exhalation undo the pose, relax in Savasana for twenty seconds in preparation for the Sit-up and Happy Cow Face.

"As you embrace the process-oriented approach instead of the outcome oriented approach, you'll achieve better results overall."- *T Sanchez*

Sit-up
1. In Savasana, become aware of your own weight, bring feet together and straighten your legs.

2. Raise both arms above your head, keep palms facing up and inhale.

3. Exhale completely and at the base of exhalation with one motion sit up, dive forward over your legs and touch toes with your hands.

25. Happy Cow Face (right &left)

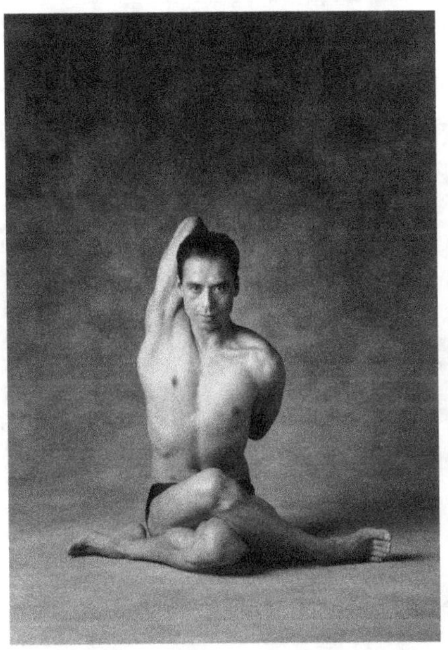 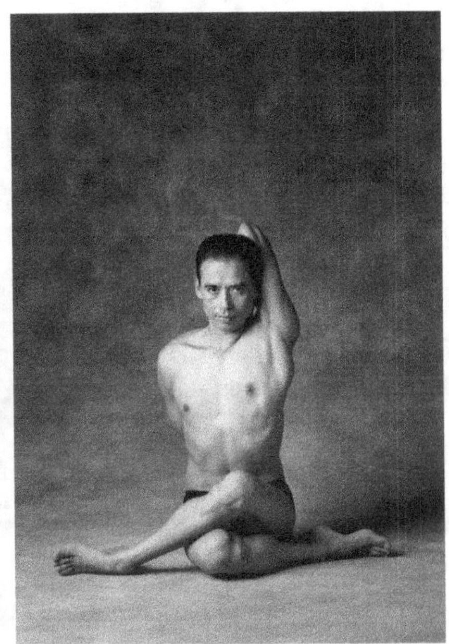

1. Kneel down Japanese style and breathe.

2. Place your hands on the floor in front of your body, and stand up on your knees.

3. Bring your right foot forward in within the Transverse Plane cross your right leg over the left leg.

4. Push your right foot back towards your left hip, overlap your right knee over the left knee, close the gap in between them as much as you can, and sit in between your heels.

5. Keep the sides of your feet on the floor, adjust your heels next to their opposite hips, straighten and align your spine with your axis, and breathe.

6. On your exhalation bring your right arm over your right shoulder, palm facing your spine.

7. Turn and bring your left arm behind you with palm facing away from your spine, and push it up towards your upper back, and breathe.

8. Move hands close to each other and if possible clasp them together.

9. Adjust your right elbow against the back of your head, straighten your spine and hold your head up.

10. Concentrate, breathe naturally and hold the posture for ten seconds.

11. Inhale. On your exhalation undo the posture and repeat it on left side exactly the same.

12. After completion of the posture relax in Savasana for ten seconds in preparation for the Sit- up and Spinal Twist.

"The only thing that will make you happy is being happy with who you are, and not who people think you are." - *Goldie Hawn*

Sit-up
1. In Savasana, become aware of your own weight, bring feet together and straighten your legs.

2. Raise both arms above your head, keep palms facing up and inhale.

3. Exhale completely and at the base of exhalation with one motion sit up, dive forward over your legs and touch toes with your hands.

26. Spinal Twist (right &left)

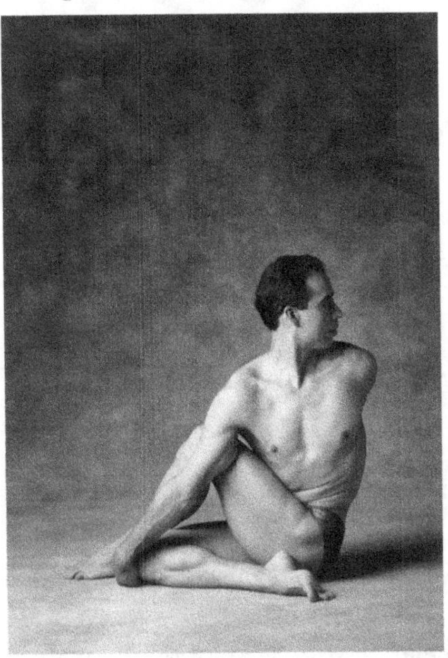

1. Sit crossed leg on your mat and breathe.

2. Bring your right knee up, place your right foot on the outside of your left knee, with toes pointing forward.

3. Flatten your right foot on the floor, and with straight spine, follow the trajectory of the Transverse Plane, and slightly turn torso and head over to your right side.

4. Bring your left arm over your right knee, place the elbow against the outside of your right leg, facing away from the knee, and stretch the arm down until you reach the knee on the floor.

5. From your wrist turn your left hand in, and if possible grab the knee on the floor.

6. Breathe, place your right hand behind you, straight your back and turn your head and torso over to your right side as much as you can.

7. Look over your right shoulder, bring right arm against your lower back and place your hand as close as possible to your left thigh.

8. Keep both buttocks flat on floor, chest up, back straight and twist torso and

head as much as you can to your right side.

9. Concentrate, breathe naturally and hold posture for twenty seconds.

10. Inhale. On your exhalation slowly undo the posture, switch legs and repeat it exactly the same on the left side.

11. Complete the posture on the left side, relax in Savasana for ten seconds in preparation for Sit-up and Kapalabhati.

"A man is as young as his spinal column". - *Joseph Pilates*

Sit-up
1. In Savasana, become aware of your own weight, bring feet together and straighten your legs.

2. Raise both arms above your head, keep palms facing up and inhale.

3. Exhale completely and at the base of exhalation with one motion sit up, dive forward over your legs and touch toes with your hands.

B. Kapalabhati (breath of fire)

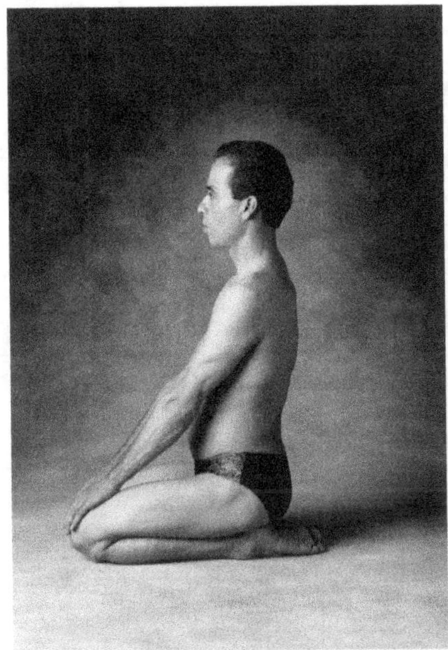 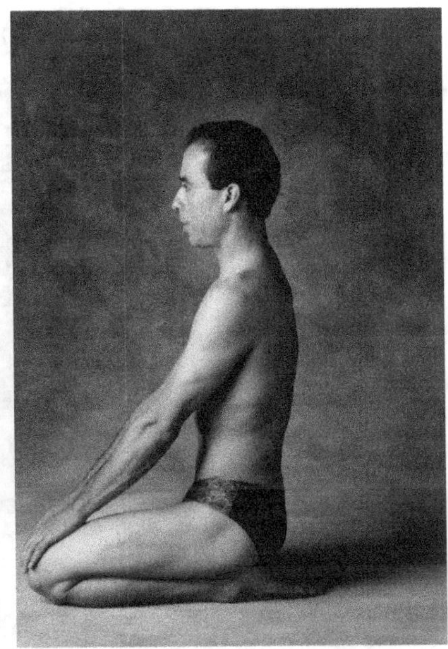

1. Sit Japanese style and place hands on their respective knees, and breathe.

2. Align your spine with your central axis, keep shoulder relaxed and hold your head up.

3. Inhale, and with an explosive exhalation through "your nose" force your breath out, then lightly relax your abdominal muscles to welcome your inhalation back in.

4. Create the explosive exhalation ½ a second apart and repeat it sixty times to complete one set.

5. Let each inhalation take place automatically, then carefully followed it with a consecutive explosive exhalation until you develop a rhythm.

6. Once the rhythm is improved increase the speed in which you do this exercise.

"The spiritual journey is one of continuous learning and purification". - *unknown*

Savasana

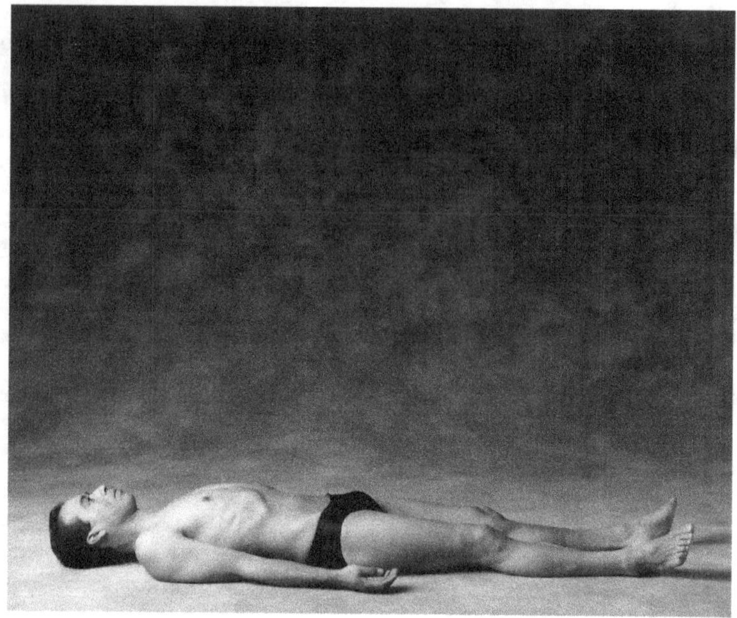

1. Lay down on your mat, face up, and breathe.

2. Keep arms close to your torso and legs close together.

3. Look up into your own head and identify your cerebral cortex (right and left brain hemispheres).

4. Follow your feeling back to your cerebellum, brain stem and to your spinal cord and finally to your peripheral nervous system and relax them.

5. Allow your arms and legs to feel tension free and heavy.

6. Focus your attention on your tail bone (coccyx) related to your first chakra, the earth chakra.

7. After a few seconds move your attention to your sacrum related to your second chakra, the water chakra.

8. After a few seconds move your attention to your lumbar spine related to your third chakra, the fire chakra.

9. After a few seconds move your attention to your thoracic region of the spine related to your fourth chakra, the air chakra.

10. After a few seconds move your attention to your cervical spine in the neck related to your fifth chakra, the space chakra.

11. After a few seconds move your attention to your pineal gland also known as the third eye chakra.

12. And from the third eye chakra move your attention to your pituitary gland and hypothalamus, associated with the Crown chakra. The pituitary gland is considered a "master gland" due to its production of hormones that control metabolism, growth, sexual maturation, reproduction, blood pressure in addition to many other vital functions. The Crown chakra represents the infinity mind. Stay and contemplate this vital centre for a few minutes and allow the benefits of the Yoga poses to take effect.

Posture modifications
These modifications should be adopted by students with special physical needs. They include imbalances, injuries, deformities or other issues with neck, shoulders, arms, back, legs or feet. If this is you, modifying the poses will help you go deep instead of just scratching the surface of the posture.

1. Lateral Half Moon (lateral flexion), modification for students with shoulder or back issues.

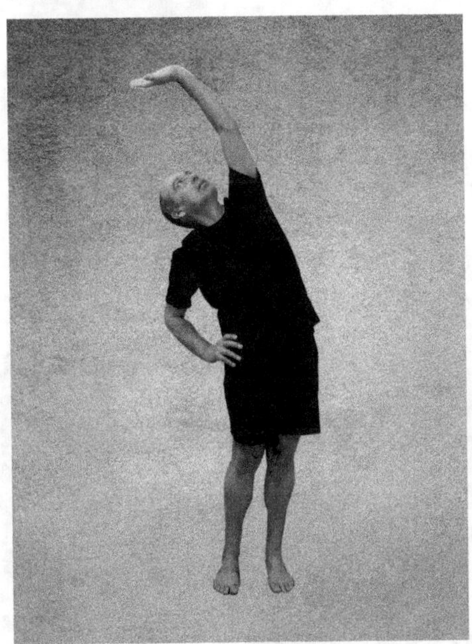

Stand in the Anatomical Position, place right hand on your right hip and stand tall, and breathe. Bring left arm above your head, turn palm up towards the ceiling and stretch. Inhale. On your exhalation follow the Coronal Plane, lean and extend your upper body, including arm over to your right side. Concentrate, breathe naturally and hold the posture for ten seconds. Return to centre and repeat exercise on the left side, after completion. Return to centre and stand in the anatomical position.

2. Back Bend (extension) modification for students with back issues.

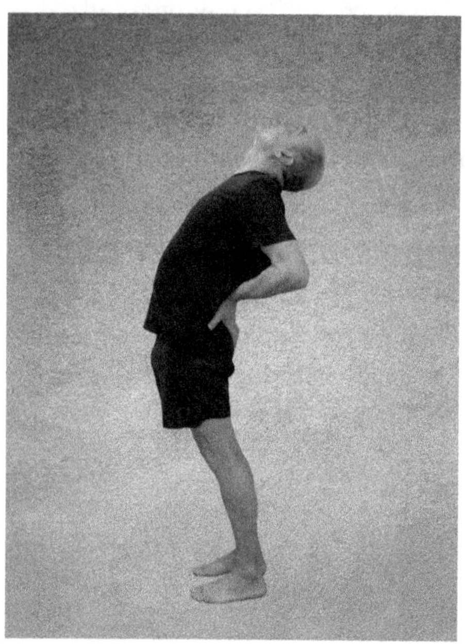

Stand in Anatomical Position, place hands on your lower back with fingertips pointing down, and breathe. Stand tall to create space in between body joints, extend your head back and focus on a point on the ceiling. Breathe and with an arched spine lean back as far as you can. Concentrate, breathe naturally and hold posture for ten seconds. Return to your standing upright position.

3. Hands to Feet (flexion) modification for students with back issues.

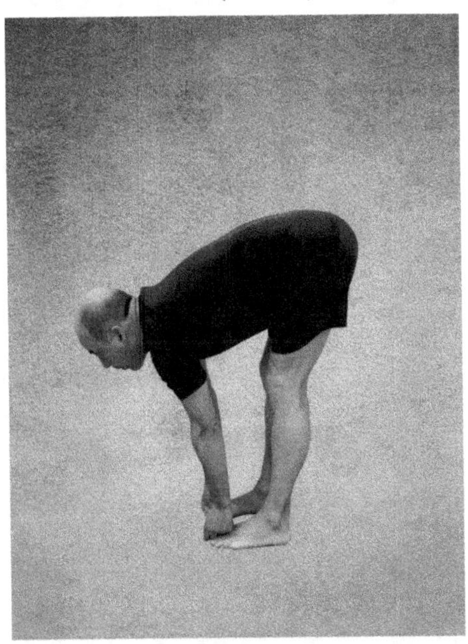

Slightly bend your knees, place hands on your upper legs, hold your head up and with the support of your hands and with a flat back bring your body down, and breathe. Lower your hand to the floor and relax your body. If possible hold your heels, keep your arms close to your calves and slowly straighten both legs. Concentrate, breathe naturally and hold the posture for twenty seconds. Inhale. On your exhalation raise your head, look forward, place hands on their respective legs and with a flat back return to your standing up right position.

4. Triangle modifications for students with back or knee issues.

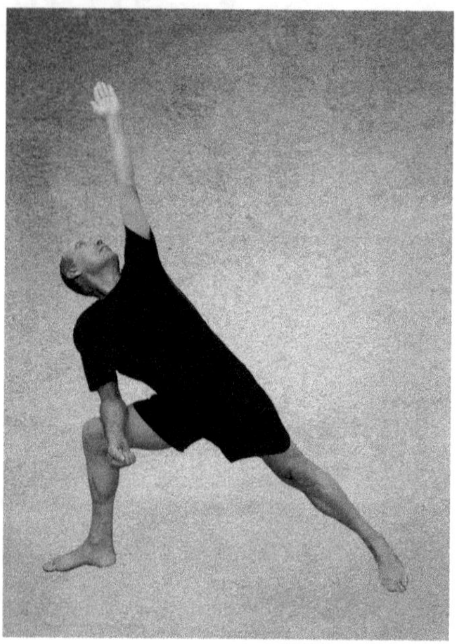

With arms above your head take a wide step to your right side and lower arms half way, parallel to with the floor, and breathe. Turn right foot to your right side and bend right knee half way. Breathe, lean over your right leg, place right elbow on your upper thigh and bring left arm straight up towards the ceiling. Align and turn head up, look at your upper left fingertips. Concentrate, breathe naturally and hold the posture for ten seconds. Inhale. On your exhalation look forward, return your upper body to centre position with leg straight and turn right foot forward. Turn left foot to your left side and repeat the pose exactly the same.

5. Standing Head to Knee modification.

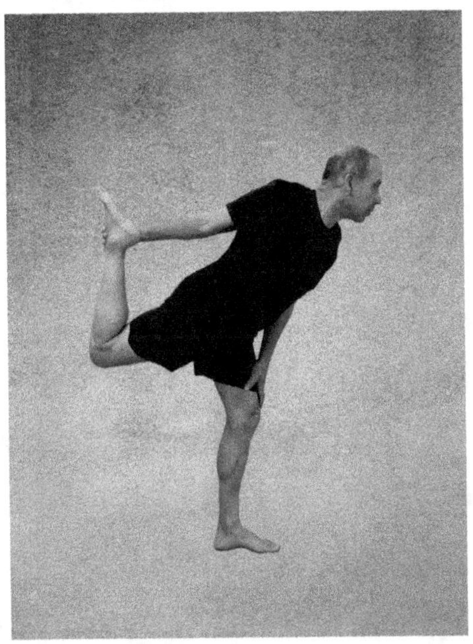

Stand tall in the Anatomical Position and breathe. Bring your right knee up towards your chest, and with interlaced fingers grab your leg two inches below your right knee. Straighten your torso, bring elbows in and ground your standing foot. Concentrate, breathe naturally and hold the posture for twenty seconds. Inhale. On your exhalation release your leg, place right foot on the floor, regroup and repeat the posture on the left side exactly the same.

6. Standing Bow modification for overweight or very stiff students.

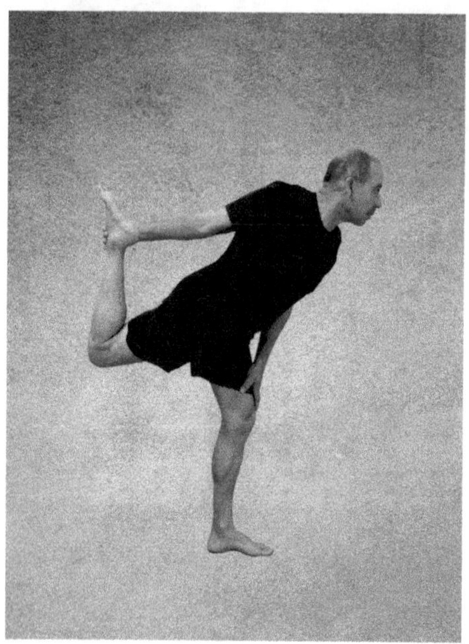

Stand in anatomical position, and breathe. Lift your right foot back towards your right hip and grab the middle of your right foot with your right hand (if possible place hand on the inside of your foot with your thumb towards your toes). Lean forward, place your left hand on your upper left th   igh for support, align hips, arch spine, lean forward even more and with pointed toes raise your right leg up as high as you can. Concentrate, breathe naturally, and hold pose for ten seconds. Inhale. On your exhalation undo the posture, stand in Anatomical Position, regroup and repeat the posture on left side.

7. Balancing Stick modification for students with back issues.

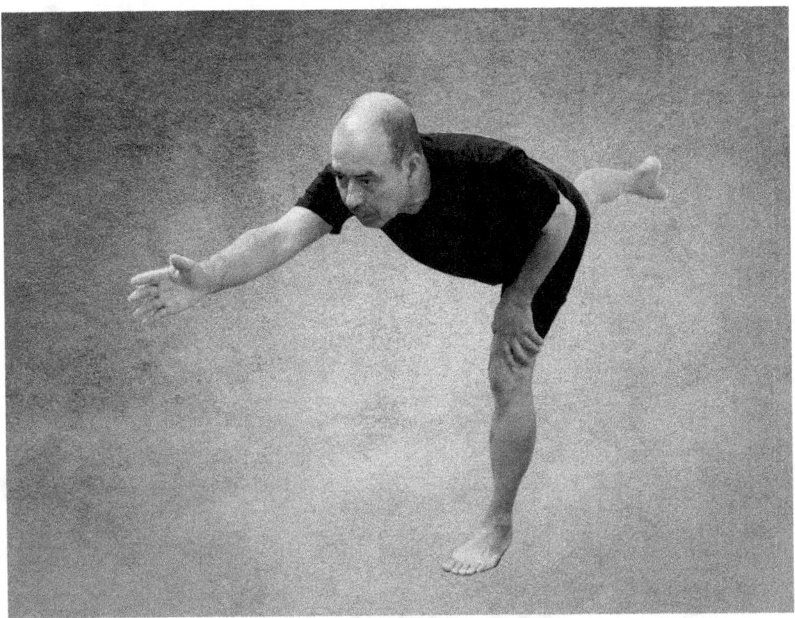

Stand in the anatomical position, and breathe. Raise both arms above your head, place palms together, cross your thumbs and stretch straight up. Inhale. On your exhalation with your right foot take a step forward and shift your weight onto your right leg.

Lean forward, as you keep your left arm extended forward place your right hand on your right thigh and lift your left leg parallel to floor. Align left hip with the floor, straighten legs, stretch left arm forward. Concentrate, breathe naturally, and hold posture for ten seconds. Inhale. On your exhalation return to starting position, regroup and repeat posture on the left side.

8. Separate Legs Stretching Head to Floor modification for students with back issues.

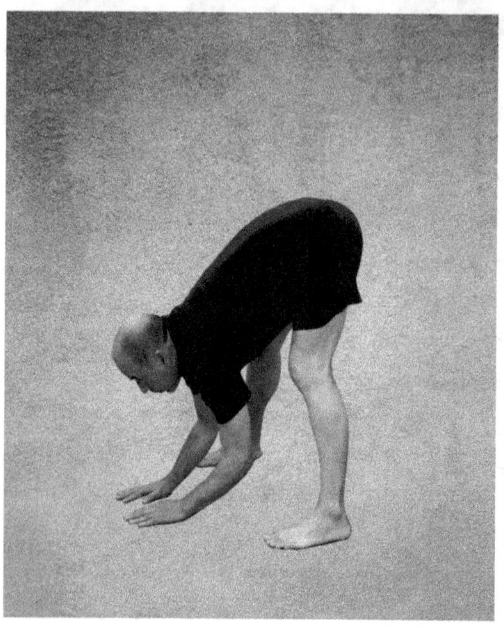

Stand in Anatomical Position, bring arms above your head, place palms together, and breathe. Take a wide step to your right side, lower arms half way and turn hand palms down. Turn your feet slightly in, place your hands on your thighs, and with a flat back stretch your upper body forward. Place your hands on the floor, bring your elbows in, and drop them down. Try to straighten your legs, and let your body hang completely relaxed. Concentrate, breathe naturally and hold the posture for twenty seconds. Return to your hands to your thighs and with a flat back stand up, bring feet together and stand in the Anatomical Position.

9. Tree modification for. Students with knee issues.

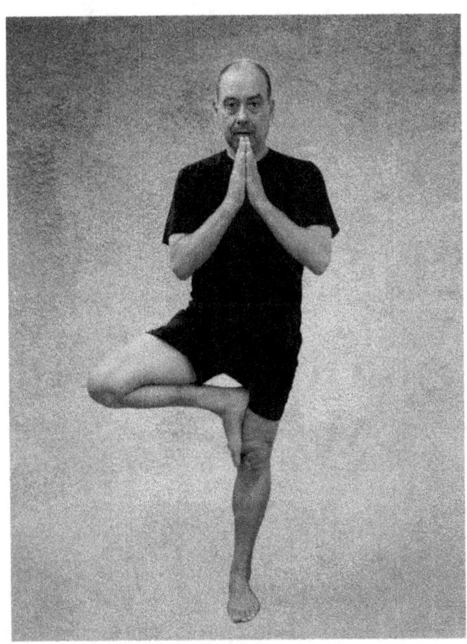

Stand tall in the anatomical position, and breathe. Raise your right knee up towards your abdomen, turn your knee out and grab your foot and place it on the inside of your upper left thigh. Adjust your right heel as close as possible to your left groin and stand straight tall. Place hands in praying position close to your heart and hold pose for ten seconds. Lower your right foot to the floor, stand in Anatomical Position, regroup and repeat the posture on left side.

10. Half Locust modification for overweight or stiff students.

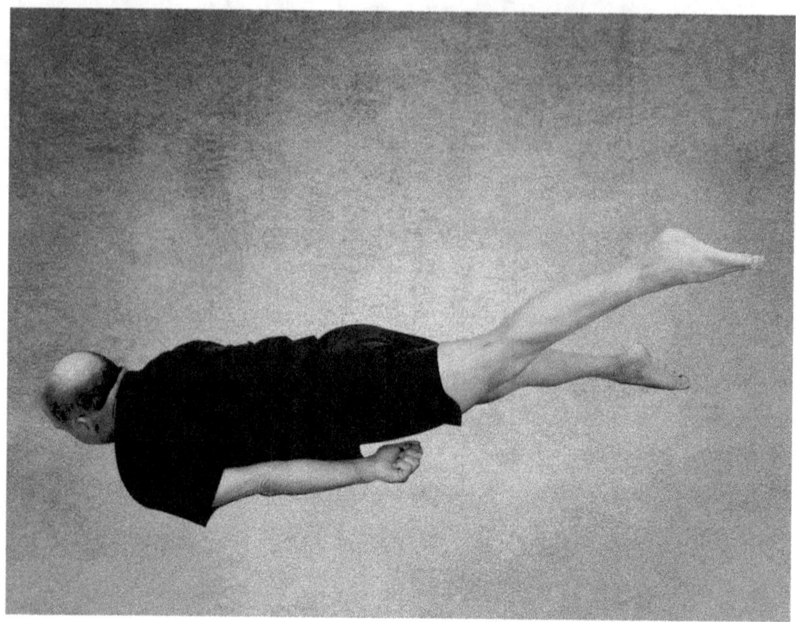

On your stomach bring arms under your body, make fists with your hands and turn them up (if not possible to bring arms under your body, keep the at your sides). Inhale. On your exhalation raise your right leg, hold the pose for ten seconds with normal breathing. Inhale. On exhalation lower your right leg and repeat the posture on the left side, exactly the same. For both legs place mouth on the floor and on your exhalation lift both legs as high as you can. Concentrate, take shallow breaths, and hold the posture for ten seconds.

11. Half Tortoise modification for students with knee or back issues.

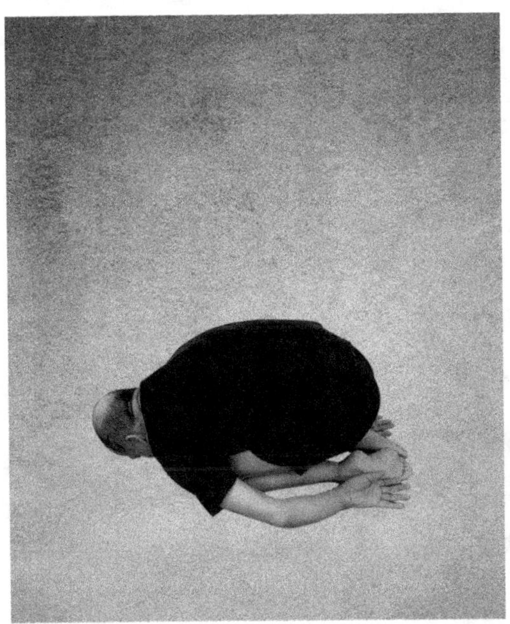

For students with knee issues, place a folded towel or pillow on your calf muscles, close to the heels, sit Japanese style and breathe. For students with shoulder issues keep arms at your sides, and lean over your thighs, place forehead on the floor and hands next to their respective hips with hand palms facing up. Concentrate, breathe naturally, and hold the posture for twenty seconds. Inhale. On your exhalation sit-up.

12. Spinal Twist modification for overweight or very stiff students.

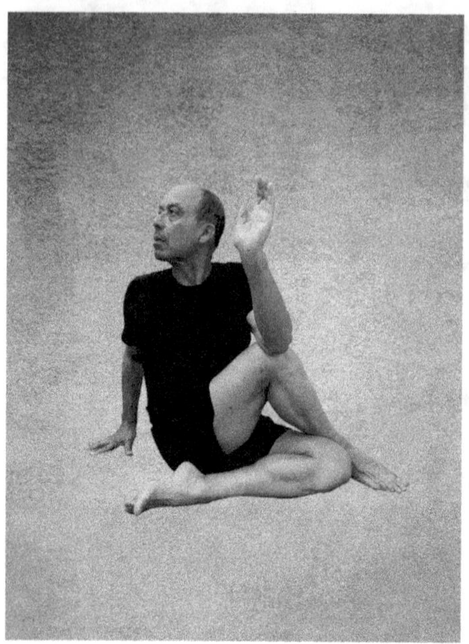

Sit with crossed or extended your legs forward, and breathe. Place your right hand on your left knee, and right hand behind you with palm flat on the floor, and your turn upper body over to your right side. Concentrate, breathe naturally and hold the posture for twenty seconds.

13. Corpse Pose modification for students with back issues.

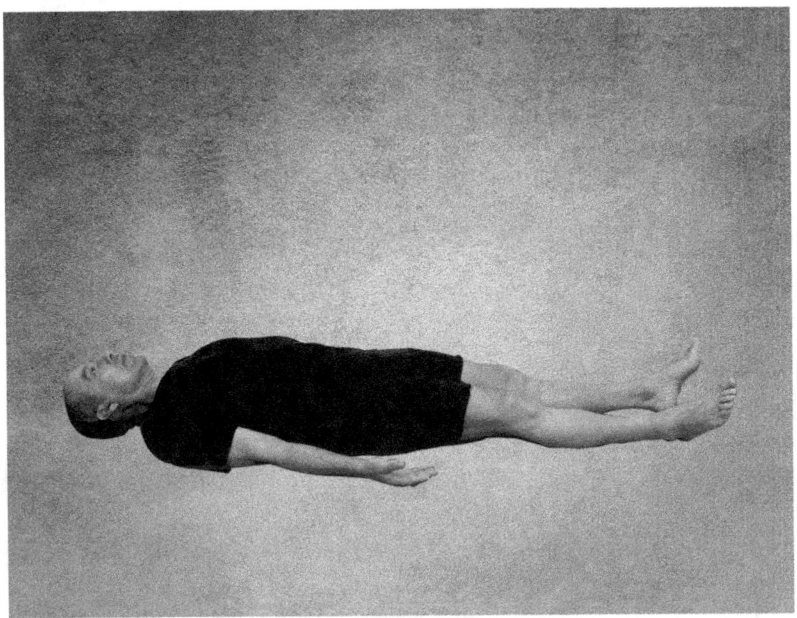

Lay down on the floor with bent knees and feet flat on the floor or place a rolled up towel or pillow under your knees. This will help relieve back tension.

THE END